EARLY ELEMENTARY CHILDREN
MOVING & LEARNING

Other Redleaf Press Books by Rae Pica

Toddlers Moving & Learning

Preschoolers & Kindergartners Moving & Learning

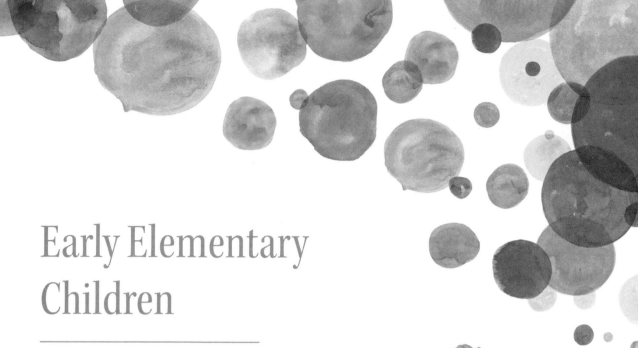

Early Elementary
Children

MOVING & LEARNING

RAE PICA

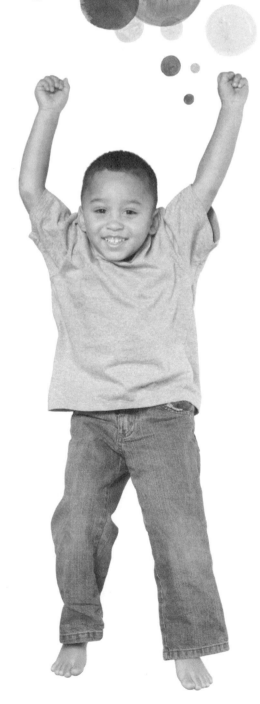

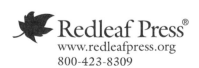
Redleaf Press®
www.redleafpress.org
800-423-8309

Published by Redleaf Press
10 Yorkton Court
St. Paul, MN 55117
www.redleafpress.org

First edition 2014
Cover design by Ryan Scheife, Mayfly Design
Cover artwork composed from images: (empty room) ssstep/iStockphoto; (watercolor circles abstract and colored spots) crisserbug/iStockphoto; (young boy playing with toy balls) jwebb/iStockphoto
Interior design by Ryan Scheife, Mayfly Design
Typeset in Kepler MM
Interior illustrations by Chris Wold Dyrud
Printed in the United States of America
21 20 19 18 17 16 15 14   1 2 3 4 5 6 7 8

Guidelines on page 12 are from *Physical Activity for Children: A Statement of Guidelines for Children Ages 5–12*, 2nd ed., by the American Alliance for Health, Physical Education, Recreation and Dance (AAHPERD) (Reston, VA: AAHPERD, 2004). Reprinted with permission.

Excerpts on page 13 are from *Developmentally Appropriate Practice in Early Childhood Programs Serving Children from Birth through Age 8*, a position statement by National Association for the Education of Young Children (NAEYC). Copyright © 2009 NAEYC. www.naeyc.org/files/naeyc/file/positions/PSDAP.pdf. Reprinted with permission.

Excerpts on pages 12 and 13 are from *NAEYC Standards for Early Childhood Professional Preparation Programs*, a position statement by NAEYC. Copyright © 2009 NAEYC. http://www.naeyc.org/files/naeyc/file /positions/ProfPrepStandards09.pdf. Reprinted with permission.

Library of Congress Cataloging-in-Publication Data
Pica, Rae, 1953-
  Early elementary children moving and learning : a physical education curriculum / Rae Pica.
    pages cm
  Summary: "This lively movement program complements any early elementary curriculum. With many developmentally appropriate, standards-based activities, this resource provides ideas for basic movement, cooperative activities, educational gymnastics, and rhythm and dance lessons" — Provided by publisher.
  Includes bibliographical references.
  ISBN 978-1-60554-269-0 (paperback)
  1. Movement education—Study and teaching (Elementary) 2. Movement education—Curricula.
3. Physical education for children.   I. Title.
GV452.P514 2014
372.86'8—dc23

                        2013031263

Printed on acid-free paper

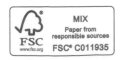

The three books in the Moving & Learning series
are dedicated to my "angel," Fredrick Davis.
He knows why.

Contents

Introduction

Unit 1

   This section consists of the "quieter" activities—those involving isolated body parts, such as the hands, face, arms, or legs, and specific relaxation exercises. Choose these activities to psychologically and physically prepare your students to begin or end their movement experiences—or any time a less vigorous activity is called for.

Unit 2

   These activities explore the fundamental locomotor and nonlocomotor skills and the movement elements of space, shape, time, force, and flow. They form the foundation of a child-centered physical education program and provide the basic knowledge essential to the next three categories.

Unit 3

   The activities in this section serve three purposes: (1) They offer the students opportunities to work cooperatively with partners and in small and large groups. (2) They provide greater challenge, beyond what the children experience in unit 2. (3) These activities can physically and emotionally prepare the students to successfully work together in those educational gymnastics and rhythm and dance activities in units 4 and 5 requiring participation in pairs or groups.

Unit 4

   Included in this section are activities related to the gymnastic skills of transferring weight, rolling, and balancing. Also included in this unit is exploration of combinations of locomotor and nonlocomotor skills, as gymnastics typically involves the sequencing of movement skills.

Unit 5

The movement element of rhythm, the musical concepts of beat and meter, and the qualities of swinging, sustained, suspended, percussive, vibratory, and collapsing movement are explored in this unit. The Statues game offers students the opportunity to improvise and express themselves to a variety of music, and the More Movement Words activities provide a chance for students to perform combinations of skills in interpretive and expressive ways. All of the activities in this unit prepare children for dance experiences in the upper elementary grades.

Acknowledgments

I couldn't be happier that the Moving & Learning series is finding a home at Redleaf Press. It's become clear to me that this is where these books belong. I'd like to thank Kyra Ostendorf and David Heath for the warm welcome, with extra-special thanks to David for being a fabulous editor. Working with you was such a pleasure!

I'm forever grateful to Richard Gardzina for the original music that accompanies these curriculum packages. He is a remarkable composer, and what I especially love about what he created here is that he never considered it "children's" music. Instead, he set out to compose and perform the best music he could.

Special thanks to the children and teachers with whom I've worked over the years—those on whom I "practiced" and those who've embraced the "movement message" at my presentations. Your enthusiasm, along with your expressions of appreciation over the years, has kept me going!

Deep appreciation to my mom, whose pride in me warms my heart.

Curriculum Connectors Charts

Openers and Closers

Activity	Art	Language Arts	Math	Music	Science	Social Studies	Page
Simon Says		X		X	X		30
See My Face					X	X	32
See My Hands					X	X	34
Mirror Game	X	X	X				36
Chanting Names		X		X			38
Relaxing Images				X	X		39
More Relaxing Images					X		40
Breath Rhythms					X		41
Punchinello	X	X		X			42
Writing in Space		X	X		X		43
Let's Focus					X		44
Blind Movement					X	X	45
Arms in Motion		X					46
Legs in Motion		X					47
Exploring Right and Left	X		X				48
Body-Halves Opposition		X			X		49
Imagining Sports						X	50
Moving As If			X			X	51
Imagining Inanimate Objects					X	X	52

Basic Movement

Activity	Art	Language Arts	Math	Music	Science	Social Studies	Page
Exploring Up and Down	X	X	X	X	X		54
Space Exploration	X		X	X	X	X	57
Body-Part Relationships	X		X		X		59
Exploring Body and Spatial Directions	X	X				X	61
Making Shapes	X	X	X				63
Directing Traffic	X		X	X			65
Moving Slow/Moving Fast		X	X	X			66
Slow-Motion Moving			X	X			68
Exploring Accelerando and Ritardando			X	X		X	69
Soft and Loud			X	X		X	71
Robots and Astronauts				X	X		73
Staccato/Legato		X		X			74
Exploring Opposites		X				X	75
Bending and Stretching	X		X				76
Exploring Bending and Stretching	X		X		X		78
Let's Shake		X		X	X		80
Let's Sway				X	X	X	82
Let's Sit	X		X				84
Let's Turn					X		85
Let's Twist				X	X		87
Let's Walk				X		X	88
Let's Run				X		X	90
Let's Jump					X	X	91
Let's Leap					X		93
Let's Gallop		X		X	X		94
Let's Hop					X		95
Let's Slide		X		X		X	96
Let's Skip		X		X			98

Cooperative Activities

Activity	Art	Language Arts	Math	Music	Science	Social Studies	Page
Bridges and Tunnels	X		X			X	102
Switcheroo!					X	X	103
Follow the Leader	X	X				X	104
Pass a Movement			X			X	106
Cooperative Musical Chairs		X	X	X		X	107
Mirror Game II	X				X	X	108
Shadow Game	X	X			X	X	109
Circle Design	X		X			X	110
Palm to Palm	X					X	112
Forming Shapes with Partners	X		X			X	113
Forming Letters with Partners	X	X	X			X	114
Touch and Move			X			X	115
Matching Shapes	X	X	X			X	116
Moving Forward with a Partner		X		X		X	117
Ducks, Cows, Cats, and Dogs	X	X	X	X	X	X	119
Synchronized Partners					X	X	120
Turning with a Partner			X		X	X	121
Footsie Rolls					X	X	122
Let's Slither					X	X	123
Exploring Contrasts		X	X			X	124

Educational Gymnastics

Activity	Art	Language Arts	Math	Music	Science	Social Studies	Page
Locomotion					X		126
Moving with Limitations			X		X		127
Jumping and Landing					X		129
Exploring Weight Placement					X		130
Counting Body Parts			X		X		131
Static Balance	X		X		X		132
Sitting Balances					X		134
Dynamic Balance					X	X	135
Let's Roll I	X		X		X		136
Let's Roll II					X		137
Symmetrical and Asymmetrical Balances	X		X		X	X	138
Balance and Recovery			X		X		139
Partner Balance					X	X	140
More Partner Balances					X	X	141
Group Balance			X		X	X	143
Exploring Upside Down	X	X	X		X		144
Discovering the Forward Roll	X	X			X		146
Combining Locomotor Skills		X					147
Movement Words		X					149
Gymnastic Sequences		X			X		150

Rhythm and Dance

Activity	Art	Language Arts	Math	Music	Science	Social Studies	Page
Body Sounds			X	X		X	152
Echoing Rhythms		X	X	X			153
Clapping Names		X	X	X			154
Pass the Beat		X	X	X			155
Rain Dance		X	X	X			156
Common Meters		X	X	X			157
A Not-So-Common Meter		X	X	X			158
Four Beats to the Measure		X	X	X			159
Ten Seconds			X				161
Let's Swing			X	X	X		162
Vibration				X	X	X	164
Percussion				X	X		165
Suspend and Collapse		X		X	X		166
More Movement Words		X				X	168
Let's Step-Hop			X	X		X	169
A Square Path			X	X			171
Exploring 3/4 Time	X		X	X			172
Zigzagging Pathways			X	X			174
The 3/4 Run	X		X	X			175
Making Dances		X		X		X	176

Song List

Title	Length	Page
"High and Low"	1:50	54
"Space Exploration"	2:40	57
"Moving Slow/Moving Fast"	2:44	66
"Slow-Motion Moving"	2:16	68
"Getting Fast/Getting Slow"	2:25	69
"Moving Softly/Moving Loudly"	2:47	71
"Getting Louder/Getting Softer"	2:31	71
"Robots and Astronauts"	3:19	73
"Staccato/Legato"	3:13	74
"Shake It High/Shake It Low"	2:58	80
"Swaying Song"	2:02	82
"Twisting"	2:02	87
"Walking Along"	1:41	88
"The Track Meet"	1:21	90
"Giddy-Up"	1:39	94
"Skipping Song"	1:09	98
"Rain Dance"	2:49	156
"Common Meters"	3:59	157
"A Not-So-Common Meter"	2:00	158
"1-2-3-4"	2:57	159
"Swing and Sustain"	1:53	162
"Vibration"	1:27	164
"Percussion"	2:06	165
"Suspend and Collapse"	1:34	166
"Step-Hop"	2:14	169
"1-2-3-Turn"	1:34	171
"The 3/4 Song"	1:53	172
"The 3/4 Run"	1:52	175

Introduction

Welcome to the Moving & Learning family! The movement program you have in your hands, *Early Elementary Children*, is intended for use with children ages six to eight years old and is being used in schools, child care settings, recreation centers, and gymnastic centers throughout the United States and in several other countries.

The program consists of activities falling under five categories: Openers and Closers, Basic Movement, Cooperative Activities, Educational Gymnastics, and Rhythm and Dance. Naturally, there is some overlap and interrelatedness between activities from one category to another. However, I chose the placement of each activity according to the category for which it seemed *most* appropriate. A brief description of each category follows:

1. **OPENERS AND CLOSERS** These activities can be used as "warm-ups" and "cooldowns" in that they are intended to physically and psychologically prepare the children to begin and end their movement education class.

2. **BASIC MOVEMENT** These activities, comprising the largest category, explore the fundamental locomotor (traveling) and nonlocomotor (nontraveling) skills and the movement elements of space, shape, time, force, and flow.

3. **COOPERATIVE ACTIVITIES** Partner and group activities fall into this category and offer children the opportunity to further develop their interpersonal skills.

4. **EDUCATIONAL GYMNASTICS** Included in this section are rolling, weight transfer, and balance activities and *combinations* of locomotor and nonlocomotor skills.

5. **RHYTHM AND DANCE** All the activities exploring the movement element of rhythm are incorporated into this section, as are those related to the movement qualities of swinging, sustained, suspended, percussive, vibratory, and collapsing movement. Combinations of skills involving *emotional content* also fall into this category.

The organization of this book gives you multiple options. If you want a movement program with a little bit of everything in it, you can pick and choose from among the sections to create your own lesson plans. On the other hand, if you prefer to do units, you can use the activities within each section (which are arranged from least challenging to most challenging) to address the specific unit you are covering. And, of course, if you're just looking for a wide variety of movement experiences to offer the children, you have a great many choices within the pages of this book.

Every activity in *Early Elementary Children Moving & Learning* includes suggestions for further exploration (you'll find more about activity extensions in the "Implementing the Program" section of this introduction), some simple questions to help you evaluate whether or not the children are meeting the activity's objectives, and Curriculum Connectors that point out ways in which the activity does or can be made to correlate with other content areas.

While it is my firm belief that the body is the most important piece of equipment in a movement program, I realize that using actual equipment can add another dimension to—and increase the challenge of—an activity. So, where appropriate, I have included Adding Equipment, offering suggestions for the use of hoops, scarves, streamers, and other props that are generally available in elementary classrooms.

Because children need opportunities to explore movement on its own, allowing them to find and use their own personal rhythms, not all of the activities in this book are accompanied by music. However, children do love music—and it does contribute much to movement experiences—so it is included wherever it makes a contribution to the learning experience. Activities using music have been marked with a musical note: (♪). The songs help promote understanding of such abstract concepts as slow and fast and help children *hear* the difference, for example, between a skip and a step-hop. They also make it possible for you to add the joy and energy of music to movement experiences without the effort of first having to locate appropriate music.

The songs that are part of this program are entirely original, having been written specifically for the activities they accompany. They expose the children to both electronic and acoustic instruments and to as many musical elements as we could manage to include. I believe in variety, and variety is what this music offers the children (and you)!

Benefits of Moving & Learning

Movement experiences in general—and in *Early Elementary Children Moving & Learning* specifically—have many benefits for children. They exercise the whole body, including the mind, and not just the muscles; they create a love of movement that should develop into a lifetime desire for physical fitness; and their success-oriented philosophy provides numerous opportunities for learning, participating, and enjoying. The following are some of their more specific benefits.

Physical Development

Perhaps the simplest and most important reason children should be allowed and encouraged to move is to develop movement skills.

Although it is commonly believed children automatically acquire motor skills as their bodies develop, maturation only means that children will be able to execute most movement skills at a low performance level. Continuous practice and instruction are needed if the performance level and movement repertoire are to increase (Gallahue and Cleland Donnelly 2003). In other words, once a child is able to creep and walk, gross-motor skills should be taught—just as other abilities are taught. Furthermore, special attention should be paid to children demonstrating gross-motor delays, as such delays will not simply disappear over time.

As Linda Carson explains, families and teachers "would not advocate learning to read or communicate by having their children enter a 'gross cognitive area' where children could engage in self-selected 'reading play' with a variety of books" (2001, 9). Similarly, engaging in unplanned, self-selected physical activities—or even a movement learning center—is not enough for young children to gain movement skills.

Why does the development of motor skills matter, when not every child will go on to become an athlete or a dancer? It matters because children who feel confident in their movement skills are likely to continue moving throughout their lives. And that's significant because of the many health problems that can be attributed to sedentary living.

Although children love to move—and adults tend to think of them as constantly being in motion—children today are leading much more sedentary lives than did their predecessors. According to Nielsen research, "Older kids (ages 6–11) clock in more than 28 viewing hours per week, primarily watching TV, but also spending close to 2.5 hours watching DVDs or playing video games, with an additional hour dedicated to the DVR and 18 minutes set aside for the VCR" (McDonough 2009). In fact, watching television is the predominant sedentary behavior in children, second only to sleeping (Kaur et al. 2003). The advent of computers and video games has also contributed to the decline in activity. A study from the Kaiser Family Foundation determined that children ages eight to eighteen are spending more than seven and a half hours a day with electronic devices (Lewin 2010)—the same number of hours some people spend at full-time jobs.

Such statistics provide cause for concern regarding children's fitness levels. Studies indicate that 40 percent of five- to eight-year-olds show at least one heart disease risk factor, including hypertension and obesity. The latter, which is on the rise, particularly among children, has been linked to television viewing (Bar-Or et al. 1998). A Canadian study determined that the blood vessels of obese children have a stiffness normally seen in much older adults who have cardiovascular disease (Science Daily 2010). Furthermore, the Centers for Disease Control and Prevention (CDC) estimates that American children born in the year 2000 face a one-in-three chance of developing type 2 diabetes, previously known as adult-onset diabetes because it was rarely seen in children (2008).

A developmentally appropriate movement curriculum, such as *Early Elementary Children Moving & Learning*, can give children the practice and

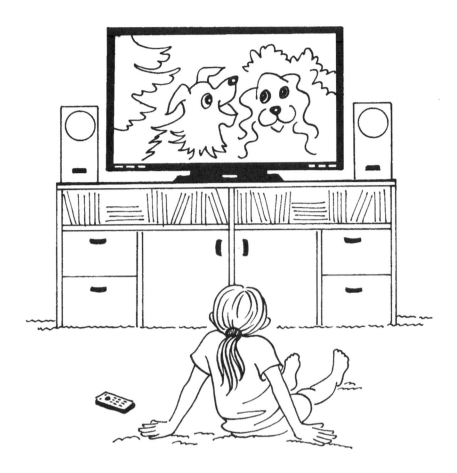

instruction necessary to refine their movement skills and expand their movement vocabularies. Moreover, with these movement activities, the children have the opportunity to frequently experience success, which makes movement pleasurable for them. Thus they are more likely to become (and stay!) physically fit.

As Eva Desca Garnet writes in *Movement Is Life*, "Our biological need for movement is ensured by the sensation of pleasure in movement" (1982, 11).

Social/Emotional Development

Marianne Frostig, in her classic book *Movement Education: Theory and Practice*, writes,

> Movement education can help a child to adjust socially and emotionally because it can provide him with successful experiences and permit interrelationships with other children in groups and with a partner. Movement

education requires that a child be aware of others in [activities] in which he shares space . . . ; he has to take turns and to cooperate. He thus develops social awareness and achieves satisfaction through peer relationships and group play. (1970, 26)

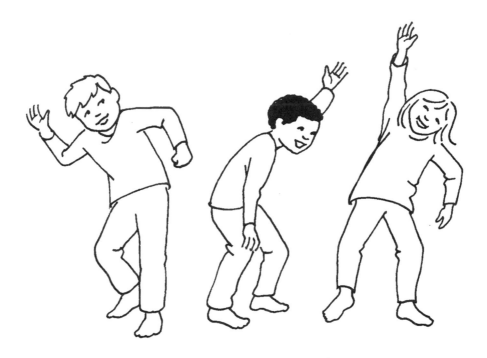

The program presented in this book provides opportunities for successful experiences, and it permits interrelationships with other children. Even before the children are asked to work with partners and groups, they must be aware of others around them, adjusting their movement patterns to avoid collisions. Of course, any time children work in pairs or in groups, as they will have an opportunity to do with this curriculum, they are learning lessons in cooperation and consideration.

The book also offers a blend of teacher-directed activities and a creative problem-solving approach to instruction. The latter lends itself to success by allowing students to respond to challenges at their own developmental levels and rates. This approach increases children's self-confidence, and thus their self-esteem, as they see their choices being accepted and praised. According to Muska Mosston and Sara Ashworth, two important results of problem solving are the "development of patience with peers and the enhancement of respect for other people's ideas" (1990, 259).

The development of *empathy* is also promoted through exposure to certain social issues that will hopefully make positive impressions in the young and open minds of your primary-grade students. For example, to physically imitate the movements and characteristics of a variety of animals is to imagine what it is like to *be* those animals. Those of us who wish to see children raised with a healthy respect and compassion for all the world's creatures can certainly hope that, once our children have imagined what it is like to be the animals, the children will never be able to imagine a world *without* them.

Cognitive Development

It has been said that joy is the most powerful of all mental stimuli. For young children, movement is certainly joyous. Beyond that, however, studies of how young children learn have proven that they especially acquire knowledge experientially—through play, experimentation, exploration, and discovery.

For example, when children move over, under, around, through, beside, and near objects and others, they better grasp the meaning of these prepositions and geometry concepts. When they perform a "slow walk" or skip "lightly," adjectives and adverbs become much more than abstract ideas. When they're given the opportunity to physically demonstrate such action words as *stomp*, *pounce*, *stalk*, or *slither*—or descriptive words like *smooth*, *strong*, *gentle*, or *enormous*—word comprehension is immediate and long lasting. The words are *in context*, as opposed to being a mere collection of letters. This is what promotes emergent literacy and a love of language.

Similarly, if children take on high, low, wide, and narrow body shapes, they'll have a much greater understanding of these quantitative concepts—and opposites—than do children who are merely presented with the words and their definitions. When they act out the lyrics to a verse like "Ten in the Bed" ("There were five in the bed, and the little one said, 'Roll over'..."), they can *see* that five minus one leaves four. The same understanding—and fascination—results when children have personal experience with scientific concepts such as gravity, flotation, evaporation, magnetics, balance and stability, and action and reaction.

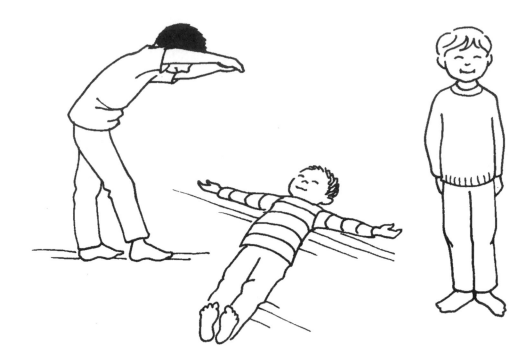

Additionally, learning by doing creates more neural networks in the brain and throughout the body, making the entire body a tool for learning (Hannaford 2005). There is a growing body of research determining that physical activity activates the brain much more so than doing seatwork. While sitting increases fatigue and reduces concentration, moderate- to vigorous-intensity movement feeds oxygen, water, and glucose to the brain, optimizing its performance.

Beyond providing an opportunity for children to "feed" their brain and to learn by doing, *Early Elementary Children* contributes to cognitive development in the following ways:

- These movement experiences offer numerous opportunities for the children to deal with the concepts of space and shape. Thus, they will be better able to deal with abstract thought. Language, numbers, and the alphabet are all abstractions, so this is very necessary preparation.
- Directionality and spatial awareness are critical to reading and writing abilities.
- By using a problem-solving method of instruction with the children, you will also be enhancing their problem-solving capabilities. They

are going to discover there will always be more than one way to
solve any problem or to meet any challenge.

- The children will experience cross-lateral movement, which helps
children cross the body's midline and activates both hemispheres of
the brain in a balanced way. Because such movements involve both
of the eyes, ears, hands, and feet, as well as core muscles on both
sides of the body, they activate both hemispheres and all four lobes
of the brain. This means cognitive functioning is heightened and
learning becomes easier (Hannaford 2005).

- Body image influences a child's emotional health, learning ability,
and intellectual performance.

Creative Development

Can you imagine a world without creativity and self-expression—not just in the
arts, but in science, business and industry, education, and life itself?

Can you honestly say you do not find some creativity in each early elementary child you work with—or that you do not know at least one adult who has
lost the ability to express himself or herself, creatively or otherwise? Where
does creativity go from the time we enter school to the time we become adults?
Is that loss of potential a result of a society and an educational system that fail
to emphasize creativity and individuality?

Why is creativity important? There are a lot of reasons. However, for young
children, creativity means there is no one right answer. This enhances their
sense of mastery, which in turn promotes their self-esteem and helps them realize they can indeed have some effect on their environment.

Teresa M. Amabile reported that the key personality traits of highly creative
people, if not naturally occurring, can be developed in childhood. These traits
include

- self-discipline about work;
- perseverance when frustrated;
- independence;
- tolerance for unclear situations;

- nonconformity to society's stereotypes;
- ability to wait for rewards;
- self-motivation to do excellent work; and
- a willingness to take risks.

(1992)

According to Mary Mayesky,

Adults who work with young children are in an especially crucial position to foster each child's creativity. In the day-to-day experiences in early childhood settings, as young children actively explore their world, adults' attitudes clearly transmit their feelings to the child. A child who meets with unquestionable acceptance of her unique approach to the world will feel safe in expressing her creativity, whatever the activity or situation. (2009, 24)

Early Elementary Children Moving & Learning encourages children to find their own ways of responding to challenges, to be individuals, and to imagine. When you meet their uniqueness with "unquestionable acceptance," the children are thus better equipped, later in their lives, to imagine solutions to problems they face, to feel empathy, and to plan futures that are full and satisfying.

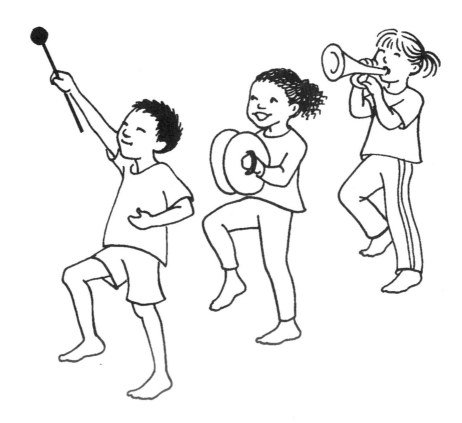

As Margaret Newell H'Doubler so aptly writes in her classic book, *The Dance and Its Place in Education,*

> as every child has a right to a box of crayons and certain instruction in the fundamental principles of the art of drawing, whether there is any chance of his ever becoming a great artist or not, so every child has a right to know how to obtain control of his body so that he may use it, to the limit of his abilities, for the expression of his reactions to life. (1925, 33)

Benefits to Children with Special Needs

All of the benefits previously cited can be applied to children with special needs. Additionally, coordination, listening skills, conceptual learning, and expressive ability are just a few of the areas enhanced through regular participation—at whatever level possible—in movement experiences.

Perhaps of greatest importance, however, is the contribution that movement experiences can make toward the special child's self-concept. Often children with disabilities fail to form a complete body image due to exclusion from physical activity. Similarly, because they do not necessarily perform the same way other children do, they develop a distorted body image (Gallahue and Cleland Donnelly 2003). Identifying and moving various body parts can "help the child discover how each body part fits into the whole schema of a human body. This enables the child to explore body boundaries and define his/her body image" (Samuelson 1981, 53). Achieving regular success in movement activities will contribute greatly to the child's confidence—perhaps offering for the first time an opportunity to feel good about himself or herself.

Another unique opportunity derived from the movement program is the chance to be part of a group. As the child's self-concept becomes more developed, he is better able to relate to others. As the child's movements and ideas are regularly accepted and valued, he receives greater acceptance from his peers. Becoming part of a group—making contributions, taking turns, following rules—has the additional benefit of enhancing social skills.

Meeting Standards

In today's educational climate, meeting standards is a consideration for all education professionals, including those in early childhood. Movement experiences in general, and those in *Early Elementary Children Moving & Learning* specifically, can address multiple standards outlined by the American Alliance for Health, Physical Education, Recreation and Dance (AAHPERD) and the National Association for the Education of Young Children (NAEYC).

For example, the position of AAHPERD in *Physical Activity for Children: A Statement of Guidelines for Children Ages 5–12* is the following:

1. Children should accumulate at least 60 minutes, and up to several hours, of age-appropriate physical activity on all, or most days of the week. This daily accumulation should include moderate and vigorous physical activity with the majority of the time being spent in activity that is intermittent in nature.

2. Children should participate in several bouts of physical activity lasting 15 minutes or more each day.

3. Children should participate each day in a variety of age-appropriate physical activities designed to achieve optimal health, wellness, fitness, and performance benefits.

4. Extended periods (periods of two hours or more) of inactivity are discouraged for children, especially during the daytime hours. (2004, 3–4)

NAEYC offers *Standards for Early Childhood Professional Preparation Programs*. Among those standards met by *Early Elementary Children* are the following:

*   Standard 1a: Knowing and understanding young children's characteristics and needs.
*   Standard 1b: Knowing and understanding the multiple influences on development and learning.
*   Standard 1c: Using developmental knowledge to create healthy, respectful, supportive, and challenging learning environments.

- Standard 3b: Knowing about and using observation, documentation, and other appropriate assessment tools and approaches.
- Standard 4a: Understanding positive relationships and supportive interactions as the foundation of their work with children.
- Standard 4b: Knowing and understanding effective strategies and tools for early education.
- Standard 4c: Using a broad repertoire of developmentally appropriate teaching/learning approaches.
- Standard 5a: Understanding content knowledge and resources in academic disciplines.
- Standard 5b: Knowing and using the central concepts, inquiry tools, and structures of content areas or academic disciplines.
- Standard 5c: Using their own knowledge, appropriate early learning standards and other resources to design, implement, and evaluate meaningful, challenging curricula for each child.
  (2009b, 11, 13, 14, and 16)

NAEYC's position statement *Developmentally Appropriate Practice in Early Childhood Programs Serving Children from Birth through Age 8* specifies that "all the domains of development and learning—physical, social and emotional, and cognitive—are important, and they are closely interrelated. Children's development and learning in one domain influence and are influenced by what takes place in other domains" (2009a, 11). The position statement instructs teachers to "plan curriculum experiences that integrate children's learning *within* and *across* the domains (physical, social, emotional, cognitive) and the disciplines (including language, literacy, mathematics, social studies, science, art, music, physical education, and health)" (2009a, 21).

Implementing the Program

A lot of flexibility has been built into *Early Elementary Children Moving & Learning*. As mentioned previously, you can either pick and choose from among the five categories to create your own lesson plans, or you can use the activities within each category to address the specific unit you are covering.

If you are creating your own lesson plans, it is best to begin by choosing an opener and closer for each lesson. You can then fill in the middle any way you like. If you are working with young students who are just being introduced to movement education, you should perhaps organize your lessons with one loco-motor activity, one nonlocomotor activity, and one activity exploring an element of movement. (Early elementary children will most likely move through these lessons more quickly than their younger counterparts.) When your students are ready to begin working collaboratively with partners and in groups, you can start including activities from the Cooperative Activities unit.

The units, like the activities within them, are in a developmental order. Not only do students first need to explore movement on their own before cooperating with others, but basic movement is also the foundation upon which educational gymnastics and an introduction to dance are built.

Although it is important to keep the developmental progression in mind as you go through the movement experiences, nobody knows your students better than you do. So don't hesitate to adapt the activities, perhaps abbreviating them or changing their order, if you feel it is better for your children. If certain activities are too advanced for your students, feel free to pass them by and return to them later; they are offered here as possibilities only.

The one suggestion I would strongly recommend is that you implement *lots* of repetition. As a teacher, you recognize how important repetition is to young children. Just because a movement activity appears only once in these lesson plans doesn't mean it is intended to be experienced only once! You should repeat activities and whole lessons as often as necessary to ensure success.

Scheduling Movement Experiences

If you are a classroom teacher, you have some decisions to make regarding the frequency of your children's movement experiences. How many will you schedule per week, and how will you use these lesson plans accordingly?

The *Moving & Learning* program is generally most effective when you can plan for a daily movement period. If you do incorporate movement activities on a daily basis, it is best to use no more than two lesson plans per week, repeating the activities from those plans throughout the week. Otherwise the children's senses will be overloaded and focusing will be much more difficult. If, on the other hand, you intend to conduct only one to three movement sessions per week, it is best to use only one lesson plan, incorporating extensions as is appropriate, during successive classes.

Finally, should you wish to adapt the lesson plans, remember that a lesson should include both large and small movements whenever possible. In most cases, this also means that the lesson will consist of both vigorous and not-so-vigorous activities, which you will definitely want to alternate, for your sake as well as the children's.

Creating a Positive Learning Environment

Success is always the goal in a *Moving & Learning* program, so the atmosphere of your class plays an important role. Managing the class must be handled with special care. With so much activity involved, however, maintaining discipline is not always easy.

But children love to move, and they like to show off and display their abilities especially to you. You can use this to your advantage when presenting challenges. If you introduce the challenges with a phrase like "Show me you can" or "Let me see you," the children will *want* to show you they can. It is a simple technique, but amazingly effective!

There are fewer behavioral problems when a program is success oriented from the beginning.

A child who is experiencing success is less likely to become bored or want to wreak havoc upon the class.

There are, however, two important rules you should explain to the children in the beginning and enforce consistently. The first is that there are to be *no collisions*. In fact, there should be no touching unless it happens to be a specific part of an activity. To phrase this positively, you can say, "We will respect one another's space," or "We will always leave room for our friends to move." At the start this may be difficult to enforce, especially with the youngest students— because they generally enjoy colliding with one another! So it is your challenge to make it a goal for the children not to interfere with one another.

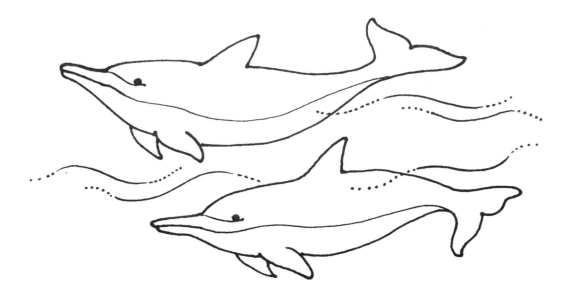

You can accomplish this by asking the children to space themselves evenly at the beginning of every movement session; carpet squares or hoops can help with this. Explain the idea of personal space to them, perhaps by encouraging the children to imagine they are each surrounded by a giant bubble; whether standing still or moving, they should avoid causing any of the bubbles to burst. Another image that works quite successfully is that of dolphins swimming. Children who have seen these creatures in action, either at an aquarium or on television, will be able to relate to the fact that dolphins swim side by side but never get close enough to touch one another. The goal, then, is for the students to behave similarly. Providing pictures of dolphins swimming together could also be helpful.

The second rule that will contribute to a manageable and pleasant environment is that there can be *no noise* (which is different from *no sound*), ensuring that your challenges, directions, and follow-up questions can be heard at all times, with no need for shouting. You can accomplish this by establishing a signal that indicates it is time to stop, look, and listen: "Stop, look at me, and listen for what comes next." Choose a signal the students should *watch* for, like two fingers held in the air, or something they must *listen* for—such as a hand clap, a strike on a triangle, or three taps on a drum—and make it their "secret code." A whistle is generally not suitable, as it can be heard above a great deal of noise, which means the children will know they can create a ruckus and still hear your signal. (In the same way that a whisper is more effective than a shout, you want a quieter signal that the children have to be *listening* for.) Nor will your voice be effective, as it is heard so often by the students.

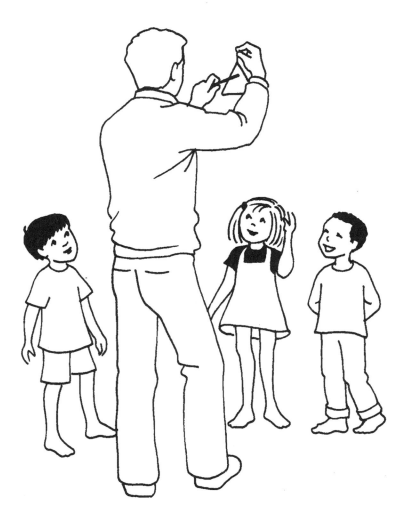

If a child still acts out, distracting or endangering other students, ask the child to sit on the sidelines and act as audience. However, give the child the responsibility of deciding when to rejoin the activities by stating, "When you are ready to join us again, let me know." Whether the child is on the sidelines by request or is simply reluctant to participate, she or he should be allowed to observe only.

In general, as in all matters relating to movement education, a positive attitude is the key.

Movement experiences should take place in a friendly, encouraging, and fun atmosphere, balanced with some basic ground rules for human behavior. This atmosphere, together with the fact that the children are experiencing success, will ensure that behavioral problems will be minimal.

Suggested Attire

Whenever possible, the children should move in unrestrictive clothing—for obvious reasons. But the most important contribution to effective movement is probably bare feet.

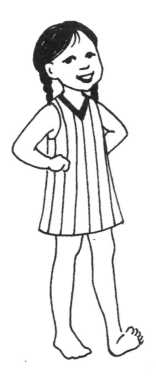

Children have worn sneakers during physical activity for so long now that we seem to have forgotten that the feet do have sentient qualities. They can grip the floor for strength and balance, and the foot consists of different parts (toes, ball, heel) that can be felt and used more easily when bare. Besides, young children feel a natural affinity for the ground, which can be enhanced by stripping away all the barriers between it and the feet.

Of course, sometimes it simply is not possible for the children to perform barefooted, as when a child is wearing tights or health regulations forbid it. If the choice becomes sneakers or stocking feet, then choose the sneakers. It is much too dangerous to move in socks or tights, even on a carpet, and sensing how easy it would be to slip will greatly restrict the child's freedom of movement.

Teaching Methods

This book employs the three teaching methods most often used in movement education: *exploration*, which should play the largest role in your students' movement experiences; the *direct approach*; and *guided discovery*, which early elementary children, due to their stage of cognitive development, are ready to begin handling.

EXPLORATION Exploration is developmentally appropriate for young children and should be the teaching method most widely used in movement programs for primary-grade children. Because it results in a *variety* of responses to each challenge presented, it is also known as divergent problem solving. For example, a challenge to demonstrate crooked shapes could result in as many different crooked shapes as there are children responding.

This approach to instruction has never been better described than by Elizabeth Halsey and Lorena Porter:

> [Movement exploration] should follow such basic procedures as: (1) setting the problem; (2) experimentation by the children; (3) observation and evaluation; (4) additional practice using points gained from evaluation. Answers to the problems, of course, are in movements rather than words. The movements will differ as individual children find the answer valid for each. The teacher does not demonstrate, encourage imitation, nor require any one best answer. Thus the children are not afraid to be different, and the teacher feels free to let them progress in their own way, each at his own rate. The result is a class atmosphere in which imagination has free play; invention becomes active and varied. (1970, 76)

In other words, you will present your students with a challenge (for example, "show me a pointed shape"), and the children will offer their responses in movement. You can then issue additional challenges to continue and vary the exploration (*extending* the activity), or you can issue follow-up questions and challenges intended to improve or correct what you have seen (*refining* responses).

Extending exploration is a technique that requires your time, patience, and practice. If you are not yet comfortable with all aspects of exploration, you may rush and hurry from one movement challenge to the next. Not only does this leave the class with too much time and nothing left to do, but it also fails to give children ample experience with the exploration process and with the movements being explored.

In addition to issuing a follow-up to "find another way," you can use the elements of movement (considered adverbs used to modify the skills, which are regarded as verbs) to extend activities. For instance, if the locomotor skill of walking were being explored, there would be a number of choices with regard to how to perform the walking: forward, backward, to the side, or possibly in a circle. The element of space is being used here. The walk could be performed with arms or head held in various positions (shape), quickly or slowly (time), strongly or lightly (force), with interruptions (flow), or to altering rhythms (rhythm).

Of course, you must design problems and suggest extensions that are developmentally appropriate and relevant to the subject matter and to the children's lives. You must also provide the encouragement children need to continue producing divergent responses. Encouragement should consist of *neutral* feedback (for example, "I see you're walking in a bent-over shape").

Although you must be careful to accept all responses, there will come a time when you wish to help the children improve, or refine, their solutions. If, for example, you have challenged the children to make themselves as small as possible and some children respond by lying flat on the floor, you should not observe aloud that this response is incorrect. In fact, it is not necessarily incorrect; it is simply another way of looking at things. However, because you want the children to truly experience a small shape, you might use the follow-up question, "Is there a way you can be small in a rounded, or curled, shape?" to encourage a different response. Although you have helped the children improve their responses, individuality is not stifled, as diverse solutions are still possible (for example, some children will make a small rounded shape in a sitting position, some will lie on their backs, others on their sides, and so on).

THE DIRECT APPROACH As children mature, they have to learn to follow directions and to imitate physically what their eyes are seeing (for example, when they must write the letters of the alphabet as seen in a book or on a board). According to Mosston and Ashworth, "Emulating, repeating, copying, and responding to directions seem to be necessary ingredients of the early years" (1990, 45). They cite Simon Says, Follow the Leader, and songs accompanied by unison clapping or movement as examples of "command-style" activities enjoyed by young children. Mirroring and fingerplays are among the other activities that they suggest fit into the same category.

With the direct approach, the teacher makes all or most of the decisions regarding what, how, and when the students are to perform (Gallahue and Cleland Donnelly 2003). This task-oriented approach requires the teacher to provide a brief explanation, often followed by a demonstration, of what is expected. The students then perform accordingly, usually by imitating what was demonstrated.

One advantage of this approach is that it produces immediate results. This, in turn, means you can instantly ascertain if a child is having difficulty following directions or producing the required response. For example, if the class is playing Simon Says and a child repeatedly touches the incorrect body part, you are at once alerted to a potential problem, possibly with hearing, processing information, or simply identifying body parts.

Mosston and Ashworth cite achieving conformity and uniformity as two of the behavior objectives—and perpetuating traditional rituals as one of the subject matter objectives—of the direct approach (1990). For example, if "rituals" like "The Hokey Pokey" are to be performed in a traditional manner, with all the children doing the same thing at the same time, the only expedient way to facilitate these activities is with a direct approach, using demonstration and imitation. Although conformity and uniformity are not conducive to creativity and self-expression, they are necessary to the performance of certain activities. Because such activities are fun for young children and can produce a sense of belonging, they should play a role in the movement program. For early elementary children, however, they should not play the largest role; that distinction should be given to exploration.

GUIDED DISCOVERY EXTENSIONS Guided discovery extensions, refining responses, and neutral feedback are also elements of the third teaching method employed: guided discovery, which, like exploration, is known as an indirect or child-centered (as opposed to teacher- or task-centered) teaching style.

With guided discovery, also known as convergent problem solving, you have a specific task or concept in mind (for example, teaching the children to perform a step-hop, or that a wide base of support provides the stablest balance).

You then lead the children through a sequence of questions and challenges toward discovery of the task or concept. This process, while still allowing for inventiveness and experimentation, guides the children as they *converge* on the right answer.

One example is a series of questions that leads the children toward discovery of a forward roll. Instead of merely *showing* the children how to perform this skill, you might issue challenges similar to the following:

- Show me an upside-down position with your weight on your hands and feet.
- Show me an upside-down position with your weight on your hands and feet and your tummy facing the floor.
- Show me you can put your bottom in the air.
- Look behind yourself from that position.
- Look between your legs at the ceiling. Try to look at even more of the ceiling.
- Show me you can roll yourself over from that position. Can you do it more than once?

Although guided discovery does take longer than the direct approach, many educators feel its benefits far outweigh the time factor. Among other benefits, with problem solving in general (convergent or divergent), the children are not only learning skills, but are learning *how* to learn. Guided discovery, specifically, enables children to find the interconnection of steps within a given task.

When using guided discovery with children, it is important to accept all responses—even those considered "incorrect." For example, if you have asked a series of questions designed to ultimately lead to the execution of a forward roll and some children respond with other rolls, these responses must also be recognized and validated. The children can then be given more time to "find another way," or the teacher can continue, asking even more specific questions, until the desired outcome is achieved.

One important tip is that the teacher should never provide the answer (Graham 2008; Mosston and Ashworth 1990). If the answer is given in the beginning, the children cannot discover it on their own. One cannot discover what one already knows. If the children do not discover the expected solution and the teacher ultimately gives the answer anyway, the children will expect this and will be less enthusiastic about exploring possible solutions themselves. Graham also maintains that because wonder and curiosity are valuable mental processes, there is no harm in concluding a lesson in which the children have yet to discover the solution (2008).

Adapting Activities

Although movement experiences entail an additional challenge for children with special needs, movement education is well suited to these children. Its philosophy and practice lend themselves to inclusion of, and success for, all children. Thus, when incorporating children with special needs into movement activities, you must be sure that your challenges can be met by all of the children.

Keep in mind that every child will be able to respond in some manner. For example, Samuelson explains that the blink of an eye, the inhalation of a breath, and the twitching of fingers are all movements (1981). Thus they can be considered responses to challenges and can even be used for demonstration purposes, with the remaining children being asked to replicate these movements. Not only does this include the child with special needs, but it also places her in what is probably an unfamiliar role—that of leader.

This book, of course, cannot do justice to the vast topic of children with special needs or cover all the different special needs that teachers and caregivers may encounter. However, the following are some guidelines for helping children with physical challenges, hearing impairments, and visual impairments achieve success.

Physical Challenges In general, a child with physical disabilities should be encouraged to participate at whatever level is possible. A child may have to substitute swaying or nodding the head for more difficult rhythmic responses. If the child cannot hold rhythm instruments, he can wear bells attached to elastics or Velcro placed around his wrists and simply *become* a musical instrument. Children in wheelchairs will have to experience locomotion on wheels rather than on foot—whether propelling themselves or being pushed by a peer.

Cane or crutch tapping can substitute for hand clapping or foot stomping, and upper-body movements can replace lower-body movements.

Movement is typically not a problem for children with hearing impairments unless there is damage to the semicircular canals. If so, the children will have balance problems, which can result in delays in motor ability. Children with such damage should refrain from taking part in potentially dangerous balance activities—for example, climbing or tumbling actions requiring rotation— unless assistance is provided.

AUDITORY CHALLENGES For all children with hearing impairments, the major challenges involved in participating in movement experiences are related to the use of music and the presentation of instructions. You can take a number of steps to help lessen the latter problem. Place children with difficulty hearing in the front of the room. Distractions like background music or others talking should be eliminated. When speaking, you should always face the child with a hearing impairment and avoid covering your mouth. You should also speak in low tones (not low as opposed to loud but low pitched as opposed to high pitched) because children with hearing impairments are better able to hear low-frequency sounds. Flicking the lights off and on is a signal that you can use to instantly get children's attention.

During music activities, remember that although a child may not be able to hear the music, she will be able to feel it. Children with hearing impairments can place their hands on the CD player or the instrument being used to make music to feel the vibrations and establish a rhythm. Lying on a wooden floor often enables children to feel the vibrations with the whole body.

Imitation is another important tool in being able to experience rhythms with and without music. Children with hearing impairments should be encouraged to imitate their peers as they clap hands, stamp feet, march, gallop, and skip.

Finally, movement experiences that meet the needs of children at all levels of ability only need minor modifications to meet the needs of children who are visually challenged. Children with visual limitations tend to rely more heavily on adults than do sighted children and often display hesitation and caution when asked to move. However, they have to their advantage auditory and tactile skills that become increasingly stronger, and these senses can be used to enhance kinesthetic skills.

VISUAL CHALLENGES When working with children with sight impairments, you have a number of methods you can use to help ensure greater success. Children with limited vision should be placed near you so they can see more easily. Holding hands with you or with a responsible partner or having a partner place his hands on the hips or shoulders of the child with visual impairments are ways of using the tactile and kinesthetic senses to encourage movement and alleviate the fear. You can also use touch to help a child achieve an appropriate shape or position.

To make use of the child's auditory sense, use verbal cues and clear, succinct descriptions when presenting challenges and when offering feedback. Statements like "You are lifting and lowering your heels to move up and down" have the additional benefit of increasing the child's body awareness. Such statements as "Everyone tilt their head side to side" help the visually impaired child realize that her body is like the other children's.

No matter what special needs a child may have, he or she can be included successfully in most movement activities.

Making Transitions

Whether the children are going on to another content area, to lunch, or home to parents at the end of your movement activities, it is always a good idea to help them wind down a bit before sending them on their way. This is where some relaxation techniques come into play.

You may be surprised to learn that relaxation plays other important roles in movement experiences other than just offering rest. Relaxation prepares children for slow or sustained movement, which requires greater control than fast movement. Being relaxed also provides children with the opportunity to experience motionlessness, giving more meaning, in contrast, to movement. Tension control can help children learn better, as stress has been found to have a negative impact on learning. Additionally, if you use imagery to promote relaxation, you will be enhancing the children's ability to imagine. If you use music, you will be exposing the children to the world of quiet, serene music. The following are some specific suggestions.

IMAGERY What comes to mind when you think of rag dolls, limp noodles, melting ice cubes, or soggy dishrags? Relaxation! Ask the children to pretend to be one of these objects, and just watch those muscles relax. Or paint a picture in their minds: Ask them to lie on the floor, imagining they are floating on a cloud or at the beach. For the latter, talk to them (softly!) about the warmth of the sun, the cool breeze, and the gentle sounds of the waves and the gulls circling overhead; and do not be surprised if a few of them drop off to sleep.

SLEEPING CONTEST If you have a particularly competitive group of children, you might find that a sleeping contest works best of all. Ask them to show you who in the class can sleep the soundest (without snoring!), and just watch as they drop to the floor! Of course, there can be no one winner, so you will have to congratulate them all on being the best sleeping class you have ever seen.

MUSIC There are lots of soothing pieces to choose from, whether with vocals or without—including classical music from the distant past (Mozart, Bach, and Chopin wrote some wonderfully soothing pieces) as well as New Age music, lullabies, or some of the many children's recordings made specifically for "quiet times."

Teaching Hints

The following suggestions are offered to help you facilitate movement experiences as smoothly as possible:

1. Always familiarize yourself with a lesson or activity, and particularly with a song, *before* trying it with the children.
2. When an activity calls for music, the lesson plan will specify this with a musical note ♪ and indicate which song on the compact disc is to be used. The Song List will help you find the song you need.

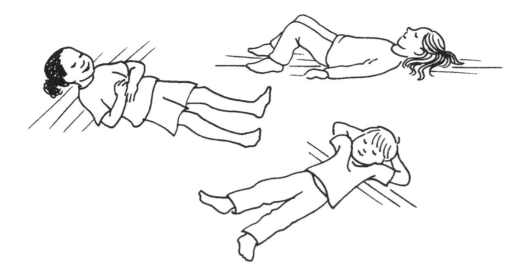

3. Discuss new or unfamiliar words or images from songs or poems with the children prior to the activity.

4. Introduce each activity to the children ("Next we're going to explore *upside-down*.").

5. Always be sure children are both familiar and comfortable with an activity before trying its extensions.

6. The lesson plans leave plenty of room for your personality and imagination. Please feel free to use them!

Early Elementary Children: Developmental Considerations

The following is some information concerning the characteristics and development of children ages six to eight years. Some of these facts are ones you are already aware of and serve here as reminders. Together with the others they will give you a better idea of what you can expect from your children as you begin this program.

1. Young children run into objects and one another because depth perception is a learned ability. Therefore, keep their paths clear for movement, and allow children enough time to change directions.

By the age of seven, children should be able to travel freely throughout a room without collisions.

2. Hand-eye and foot-eye coordination are difficult for children at the young end of this age spectrum due to slow reaction time. It is not until the age of nine or ten that they are fairly well established.

3. Fundamental movement abilities are usually present by five years of age; by the age of six, children are able to perform most locomotor skills in a mature pattern.

4. A desire to excel begins in the second and third grades; children in these grades like to be admired for doing things well.

5. By the age of eight, the child's self-concept is becoming established, but positive reinforcement from adults is still necessary for the continued development of a positive self-concept.

6. Physiologically, girls are about a year ahead of boys in their development.

7. Boys and girls share similar interests at the beginning of this age range, but interests begin to diverge toward the end.

8. First-grade children may tire suddenly, but they recover quickly.

9. Self-consciousness tends to become more of a factor toward the end of this age span.

10. Six- to eight-year-olds generally can execute two or more skills concurrently—for example, running and catching.

11. Six- to eight-year-olds can learn simple folk and partner dances.

According to Bruce A. McClenaghan and David L. Gallahue, "If a child fails to develop efficient patterns of movement during the early childhood period, he or she finds it increasingly difficult with each advancing year to acquire mature patterns" (1978, 11). Your role, therefore, is a critical one. Although you will primarily be using exploration as a teaching method, you must still be aware of how *well* the children are performing movement tasks. Also, be aware that your children will first perform each new skill in imperfect, individual ways; you should be concerned only if a child shows no progress toward mastering it after faithfully practicing the skill for a long period of time.

UNIT 1

Openers and Closers

This section consists of the "quieter" activities—those involving isolated body parts, such as the hands, face, arms, or legs, and specific relaxation exercises. Choose these activities to psychologically and physically prepare your students to begin or end their movement experiences— or any time a less vigorous activity is called for.

Simon Says

This is an excellent body-parts activity that is familiar to most children. In this activity, Simon Says is played without the elimination process. (In the traditional game, the children who need to participate the most are usually the first to be eliminated!) Begin by saying "Simon says" before each request.

"Simon" might make the following requests:

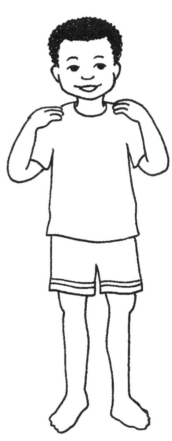

- Raise your arms.
- Touch your head.
- Stand up tall.
- Touch your toes.
- Touch your shoulders.
- Pucker up your mouth.
- Stand on one foot.
- Place your hands on hips.
- Bend and touch your knees.
- Close (open) your eyes.
- Reach for the sky.
- Give yourself a hug!

Extending the Activity: To incorporate listening skills into the activity, as with the traditional game, begin saying "Simon says" only before *some* of the requests, reminding children they are not supposed to move without Simon's permission. To keep all children participating all the time, divide the group into two circles or lines. When a child moves without Simon's permission, he or she simply leaves his or her line or circle and goes to the other.

You can also make the game more challenging by incorporating more "difficult" body parts, like elbows, wrists, ankles, temples, and shins. Additionally, the more adept your children become at the game, the faster your pace should be!

Observation and Evaluation: Can the child appropriately identify body parts? Does the child exhibit listening skills?

Curriculum Connectors: Body-part identification falls under the heading of *science* for young children, while listening skills are required in both *music* and *language arts*.

See My Face

Sit with the children and explain how they are going to discover the many different things they can do with their faces alone. Then present the following challenges to them:

- Let me see a smile; a frown.
- Make a "growling" face.
- Close your eyes real tight; open them wide.
- Wiggle your nose.
- Close your mouth real tight; open it wide like a tunnel.
- Show me you can make your mouth move from side to side.
- Pucker up like you have just sucked on a sour lemon.
- Blink your eyes open and shut like a light going on and off.
- Lick your lips like you just saw something yummy to eat.
- Show me a surprised face; an angry face; a really sad, about-to-cry face; a happy face!

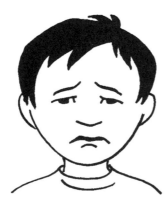 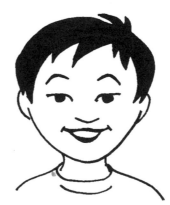

Extending the Activity: Play a game of Pass a Face. Sit in a circle with the children and begin by making a face that you "pass" to the child to your right or left. That child makes the *same* face and passes it along in the same direction. When the face has been passed all around the circle and comes back to you, repeat the process with a different facial expression.

You can make the activity more challenging by having each child imitate the face passed on to her or him, but then also making a *new* face, which she or he then passes to the next child.

Observation and Evaluation: Does the child properly identify and move facial body parts? Does the child identify with the imagery used? Can the child express himself or herself? Does the child physically replicate what the child is seeing in the activity extension?

Curriculum Connectors: Body-part identification and experiences fall under the heading of *science* for young children, while opportunities for self-expression constitute *social studies*, as does the cooperative nature of the extension activity.

See My Hands

Ask the children to sit and move their hands and fingers in the following ways:

- stretch hands and fingers as wide as possible; bend them into tightly clenched fists
- move fingers in and out very fast; very slowly
- bring hands together with much force (as though to clap them) but not letting them touch
- repeat the previous movement, with hands up high; to one side; the other side
- bring hands together using little force (making movement soft and light)
- clasp hands together and move them up and down; in and out; side to side
- turn hands from front (palms) to back
- make circles with hands without moving arms

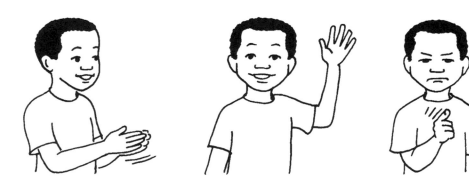

Extending the Activity: Incorporate imagery to demonstrate just how many things the hands are capable of doing and saying. Before beginning, emphasize that there is to be no touching—that they are to perform these actions "in the air." Then ask the children to show you these things:

- praying hands
- how their hands would look if they were frightened; happy; mad
- a slapping motion (as at a mosquito)

- pushing; pulling
- clapping
- beckoning
- patting
- scolding
- fanning
- writing
- painting
- playing piano; guitar; trombone
- directing traffic
- how many ways they can wave good-bye

Observation and Evaluation: Does the child have the control necessary to perform the initial activities? Can the child accurately respond without demonstration? Does the child relate to the imagery involved?

Curriculum Connectors: Becoming familiar with the capabilities and limitations of body parts constitutes *science* for young children. Role playing and the expression of emotions fall under *social studies*, as children learn about themselves and the world around them.

Mirror Game

As part of their development, children must learn to physically imitate what they experience visually. This game gives them the opportunity to do just that.

Stand where all of the children can easily see you. Explain that they should pretend to be your reflection in a mirror, imitating your every move. Then move parts of your body in various ways (for example, raising and lowering an arm, tilting your head) slowly and without verbal instruction; and the children do likewise.

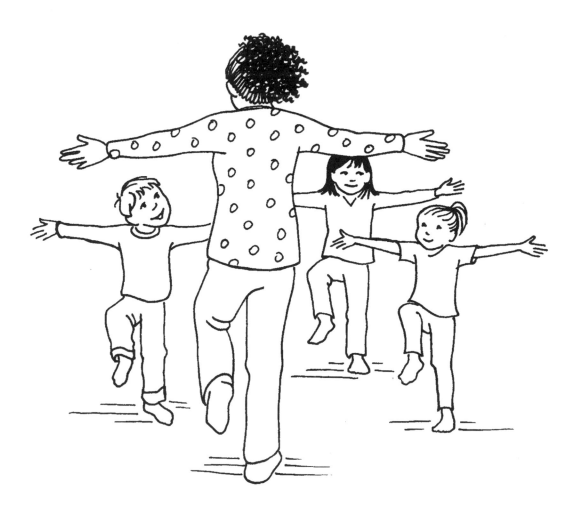

Extending the Activity: Perform a short *sequence* of movements at a slow to moderate tempo, which the class must then imitate. An example would be this: bend knees—straighten—place hands on hips.

Here are other possible sequences:

- bend knees—straighten knees
- rise on tiptoe—lower heels—clap hands twice
- bend forward at waist—straighten—place hands on head
- jump twice in place—open and close mouth—shake arms

To make the activity more challenging, all you have to do is add to each sequence! The following show the above sequences with two more steps added. Start by adding just one:

- bend knees—straighten knees—place hands on hips—nod the head—circle arms
- rise on tiptoe—lower heels—clap hands twice—turn around—clap three times
- bend forward at waist—straighten—place hands on head—jump once in place—blink three times
- jump twice in place—open and close mouth—shake arms—shake whole body—collapse to floor

Observation and Evaluation: Is the child able to imitate what her or his eyes are seeing? Is the child able to remember a sequence?

Curriculum Connectors: Being able to physically replicate what the eyes are seeing is a central component of *art*, and is necessary in learning to write (*language arts*). Sequencing is part of *mathematics*.

Chanting Names

Sit in a circle with the children and begin to slowly beat your hands on the floor, asking the children to join in. Starting with your own name, go around the circle chanting everyone's name four times, fitting the name to the rhythm of the beating.

Extending the Activity: Once children have mastered the above, pick up the tempo, chanting each name only twice.

Observation and Evaluation: Does the child maintain a steady, unhurried beat? Is the child able to rhythmically chant the names?

Adding Equipment: Instead of beating hands on the floor, the children can each hold one or two rhythm sticks.

Curriculum Connectors: Rhythm is an essential component of *music* and *language arts*, the latter because words have rhythm and individuals must develop an inner sense of rhythm when reading and writing.

Relaxing Images

Imagery can be helpful in creating relaxed bodies. Challenge children to show you what they would look like if they were soggy dishrags or jellyfish, and just watch those muscles relax! You can also invite them to imagine themselves as uncooked, cooking, and cooked spaghetti.

Extending the Activity: To help children experience the contrast between contracting and releasing muscles, challenge them to first be statues and then rag dolls. Alternate these two images, remembering to end with the rag dolls!

Another possibility is to paint a picture in the children's minds. Ask them to lie on the floor, imagining they are at the beach. Talk to them (softly!) about the warmth of the sun, the cool breeze, the gentle sounds of the waves, and the gulls circling overhead. What else might they feel and hear?

Observation and Evaluation: Does the child relate to the imagery used? Does the child demonstrate the difference between contracting and releasing the muscles? Is the child able to enter into a relaxed state?

Curriculum Connectors: Relaxation (and contraction) of the muscles falls under the heading of *science*. Playing soft, soothing *music* can also contribute to the children's ability to relax.

More Relaxing Images

To promote deep breathing, ask the children to expand (by inhaling) and contract (by exhaling) like balloons, alternately (and slowly) inflating and deflating. Children should inhale through the nose and exhale through the mouth.

Extending the Activity: "Melting" is another effective slow-motion exercise. Challenge children to imagine themselves as ice cream cones or ice sculptures slowly melting in the sun. Children also love to pretend they are the witch from the *The Wizard of Oz*, calling out "I'm melting!" as they sink to the floor.

Observation and Evaluation: Is the child able to move *slowly*? Can the child enter into a relaxed state?

Adding Equipment: Demonstrating inflation and deflation with an actual balloon can be helpful in getting the idea across.

Curriculum Connectors: Inflation, deflation, melting, and a focus on the breathing process all qualify as *science* experiences.

Breath Rhythms

Instruct the children to make a huge body shape by breathing in slowly and letting the body "grow" as they inhale. They then slowly exhale, curling themselves in toward the body center as they do.

Repeat this until the children have grasped it, and then pick up the pace. Ask your students to make the large and small body shapes more quickly by breathing in and out more quickly. Finally, you can ask them to make the large shape quickly and the small shape slowly, and then the reverse.

Extending the Activity: Challenge the children to breathe, moving out and in as though against some resistance, first exerting a lot of force and then just a little. Another alternative is to ask them to move out and in with three or four sharp accents so they are breathing in and out with short sniffs. (*Note:* To avoid hyperventilation, keep this activity short!)

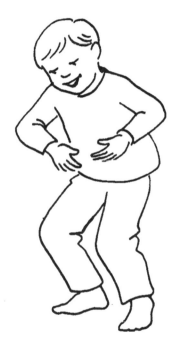

Observation and Evaluation: Does the child have the control necessary to breathe slowly? Is the child able to make the large and small shapes quickly? With varying amounts of force? Does the child understand the concept of accents?

Curriculum Connectors: Asking children to focus on their breath constitutes *science*. You can take it further by initiating a discussion about the lungs and/or by having them monitor their heartbeats throughout the exercise.

Punchinello

This activity provides an excellent review for the end of class. The children form a circle, with one child in the center (Punchinello), and chant or sing: "What can you do, Punchinello, funny fellow? What can you do, Punchinello, funny you?" The child in the center chooses one of the day's activities to demonstrate. Then the group sings: "We can do it too, Punchinello, funny fellow. We can do it too, Punchinello, funny you." And they do!

Extending the Activity: To make the activity more challenging, the child in the center can demonstrate both the activity shown by the previous Punchinello and one of his or her own, both of which the other children must also imitate. This works the memory a bit and also provides additional practice with each skill demonstrated.

Observation and Evaluation: Can the child think of an activity to demonstrate? Does the child perform the activity correctly? As a member of the responding group, does the child correctly imitate what has been demonstrated?

Curriculum Connectors: The song/chant and its lyrics qualify this activity as both *music* and *language arts*. The ability to physically replicate what the eyes see is essential to *art* and to learning to write, which provides another element of language arts.

Writing in Space

Ask the children to each choose a number, letter, word, or name that they would like to write, then write it in the air in front of them using their dominant hand. Can they do it with the other hand? Continue in this manner with a variety of numbers, letters, and words.

Extending the Activity: Ask the children to make each letter or number larger and smaller, then to display both printed and cursive letters. Also challenge them to "write" with the following body parts:

- an elbow
- a knee
- the top of the head
- the nose
- a foot; the other foot

Observation and Evaluation: Does the child accurately demonstrate the straight, curving, and angular lines of letters and numbers? Can the child show both printed and cursive letters, in both large and small sizes? Is the child able to use the designated body parts appropriately?

Adding Equipment: Children may be helped by first being able to visually track their movements. Holding a brightly colored scarf or a short ribbon stick in the hand while writing can help with this.

Curriculum Connectors: A focus on letter and number recognition constitutes both *language arts* and *mathematics*, while body-part awareness falls under the heading of *science*.

Let's Focus

This activity requires the children to isolate head movement and to use their imaginations to the maximum if they are to vary their responses.

Ask the children to focus their gaze as if doing the following:

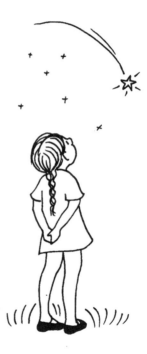

- searching for something small in a rug
- looking out a car window
- trying to see in a dark room
- watching a falling star
- watching a parade
- being hypnotized by a swinging object
- looking through a telescope
- watching a tennis game
- looking at an airplane
- watching a race

Extending the Activity: With the children in pairs, one partner moves all around the room, while the other maintains a constant focus on him or her. After a while, partners reverse roles.

Observation and Evaluation: Does the child relate to the imagery used? Is the child able to concentrate to the extent required? Can the child isolate the head's movements from the rest of the body?

Curriculum Connectors: By focusing on the sense of sight, this activity qualifies as a *science* experience.

Blind Movement

In this activity, the children are going to find out just how different familiar movements can feel when they close their eyes. Ask the children to perform the following with their eyes closed:

- touching the pointer finger to the tip of the nose
- standing on tiptoe
- standing on one foot (flat)
- leaning in all four directions
- swaying

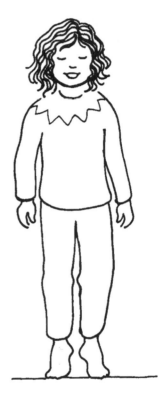

Extending the Activity: When the children are ready, challenge them to try taking a step or two—forward, sideways, and backward—with their eyes closed.

Observation and Evaluation: Does the child keep both eyes closed? Is the child able to maintain balance? Is the child afraid to move with eyes closed?

Adding Equipment: Holding a hoop around the waist can make moving "blind" feel more secure—and fun. Children will know that if their hoop touches someone else's, it's time to change directions. Make it a game of gentle bumper cars!

Curriculum Connectors: Focusing on the sense of sight, or lack thereof, places this activity under the heading of *science*. The cooperation involved in the activity using hoops brings in *social studies*.

Arms in Motion

• •

Ask the children to sit, and explain that they are going to experiment with how many ways they can move their arms alone. (*Note:* Because arms tire easily, you may have to include "resting" arms often.)

Have the children move both of their arms in the following ways:

- slowly
- softly
- quickly
- forcefully
- sharply
- in a circular manner
- swinging
- in straight lines

Extending the Activity: Challenge the children to move first the right arm (or, one arm) and then the left arm (the other) in the ways listed above. After they have had ample experience with this, ask them to move one arm in one of the ways listed above, and then to move the other arm in the *opposite* way (for example, strongly and lightly; quickly and slowly).

Observation and Evaluation: Is the child able to isolate the arms from the rest of the body? Can the child move the arms in the designated ways? Can the child isolate one arm from the other?

Adding Equipment: Holding a brightly colored scarf in each hand can make these activities more fun and visually appealing, and can also help children see the different responses better.

Curriculum Connectors: Because most of the ways in which you have asked the children to move their arms involve the use of descriptive words, these exercises, including the one exploring opposites, can be considered experiences in *language arts*.

Legs in Motion

In this activity, you will issue the same challenges presented in Arms in Motion, but the children will respond with their legs only. Therefore, they will have to be either sitting down or lying on their backs.

Have the children move their legs in the following ways:

- slowly
- softly
- quickly
- forcefully
- sharply
- in a circular manner
- swinging
- in straight lines

Extending the Activity: As you did with Arms in Motion, challenge the children to move first the right leg (one leg) and then the left (the other) in the ways listed above. After they have had ample experience with this, ask them to move one leg in one of the ways listed above, and then to move the other leg in the *opposite* way (for example, strongly and lightly; quickly and slowly).

Observation and Evaluation: Is the child able to isolate the legs from the rest of the body? Can the child move the legs in the ways indicated? Can the child isolate one leg from the other?

Curriculum Connectors: The exploration of these descriptive words, as well as opposites, constitutes *language arts*.

Exploring Right and Left

Here the children are simply going to be introduced to *laterality* (preference or dominance of using the left or right side of the body) by experimenting with movements performed on one side of the body that are imitated on the other side.

Stand facing the children, and tell them when they are working with their right and left sides, but use your opposite side to act as a mirror reflection.

Suggest the following movements (remembering to repeat them on both sides):

- Raise and lower your right/left arm.
- Move your right/left arm in a smooth, wavy way.
- Lift your right/left leg forward and then put it back on the floor.
- Lift your right/left leg to the side and put it back.
- Wiggle the fingers of your right/left hand in the air.
- Cover your right/left eye with the hand on that side.
- Cover your right/left ear with the hand on that side.
- Touch your right/left shoulder.
- Bend your right/left knee.
- Put your right/left hand on your hip on that side.

Extending the Activity: The next time you perform this activity, do not do the movements with the children.

Observation and Evaluation: Does the child appropriately identify body parts? Is the child able to isolate one side from the other?

Adding Equipment: Some physical education suppliers offer vinyl feet cutouts labeled right and left. Placing a pair of these in front of each child can help her or him see which side of the body is being used.

Curriculum Connectors: Positional concepts, like left and right, are a component of geometry (*mathematics*) and *art*.

Body-Halves Opposition

Asking separate halves of the body to perform opposite tasks is difficult for people of all ages, even when those tasks are not being performed at the same time. However, if the children you are teaching have had enough body and spatial awareness at this point, give it a try.

Have the children sit. Explain that the right side of the body can do something separate from the left side, and the top part of the body can do something separate from the bottom.

Then pose the following challenges:

- Make a slow movement with one arm and then a fast movement with the other. (Then reverse sides.)
- Show me you can make a gentle, light movement with one arm and then a strong, hard movement with the other. (Then reverse sides.)
- Make a slow, light movement with your arms and hands, followed by a fast, hard movement with your legs and feet.

Extending the Activity: Additional challenges might include the following:

- Make your head move fast and then one foot move slowly.
- Show me you can make the other foot move fast and then your head move slowly.
- Stretch the top half of your body while also bending the lower half.

Observation and Evaluation: Does the child seem to understand the concept of body-halves opposition? Is the child capable of performing the tasks?

Curriculum Connectors: Experimentation with the limitations and capabilities of the body and its parts falls under the heading of *science* for young children. Also, discussion of and experience with opposites constitutes *language arts*.

Imagining Sports

Ask the children to show you, as realistically as possible, how they would move if they were participating in a variety of sports. Individual responses will of course be based on the role or position the child has chosen to play within each sport and on her or his interpretation of how that role is played.

You might choose from the following sports:

- football
- gymnastics
- baseball
- basketball
- hockey
- golf
- swimming
- soccer
- tennis
- volleyball

Extending the Activity: Once children have portrayed one role for each sport, encourage them to find another, or to find a different way to portray the original role. You might also challenge the children to show you their movements in slow motion, as though in instant replay, and in fast forward.

Observation and Evaluation: Does the child demonstrate realistic movements for each sport? Does the child's movement remain realistic when slowed down or speeded up?

Curriculum Connectors: A discussion about the people who make their living in these sports—and the role playing—link this activity to *social studies*.

Moving As If

Stressing realism, ask your students to move as if in the following situations:

- caught in something very sticky
- taking a cold shower
- being tickled by a feather
- inside a small box
- inside a beach ball

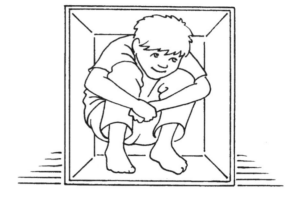

Extending the Activity: Suggest additional scenarios for each of the above. For example, if children demonstrate only *feet* caught in something sticky, encourage them to think of how it would look if other body parts were caught.
What if a foot, a hand, or a nose were being tickled by a feather? What if, while inside a small box or beach ball, they were on their bottoms, their feet, or their knees?

Observation and Evaluation: Does the child identify with the imagery used? Does the child show an ability to imagine?

Curriculum Connectors: These activities provide ample opportunity for self-expression, which comes under the heading of *social studies* for young children. The concept of *inside* is a positional word and part of early geometry (*mathematics*).

Imagining Inanimate Objects

Tell the children they are really going to have to use their imaginations for this exercise. Then ask them to show you, with their bodies, what they would look like if they were the following:

- a stapler
- a paper clip being slipped over some papers
- an ice cube melting
- a cloud drifting across the sky and slowly changing shape
- a rubber ball bouncing on the ground
- a boat being tossed by waves
- an arrow being shot through the air
- smoke coming from a chimney
- a balloon deflating

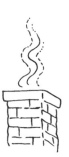

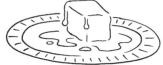

Extending the Activity: More challenging images might include the following:

- an orange being peeled
- a shirt tumbling in the dryer
- a pencil being sharpened
- a tire jack lifting a car
- a can being opened

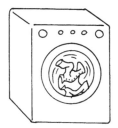

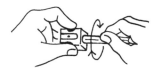

Observation and Evaluation: Does the child identify with the imagery used? Does the child demonstrate an ability to imagine?

Curriculum Connectors: Incorporate a discussion about some of these items (for example, smoke coming from the chimney, a cloud drifting and changing shape) to tie this lesson to *science*. Also, self-expression is central to early *social studies*.

UNIT 2

Basic Movement

These activities explore the fundamental locomotor and nonlocomotor skills and the elements of movement: space, shape, time, force, and flow. They form the foundation of a child-centered physical education program and provide the basic knowledge essential to the next three categories.

Exploring Up and Down

· ·

♪ "High and Low" (Length 1:50)—CD Track 1

For this initial exploration of the levels in space, pose the following questions and movement challenges:

- Show me with your body what "up" and "down" mean.
- Show me you can make your body go all the way down. All the way up.
- How high up can you get?
- Show me you can go down halfway.
- Make yourself so tiny I can hardly see you.
- Show me you can become as huge as a giant.
- Now pretend your feet are glued to the floor. Move your body up and down without moving those feet.

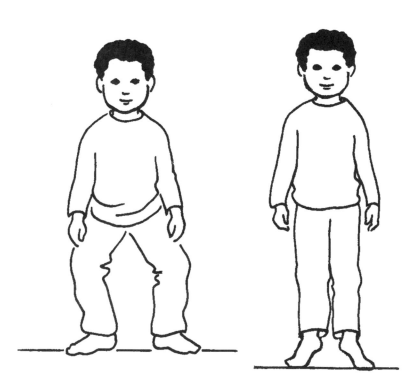

Extending the Activity: Incorporate imagery into the exploration of up and down by posing the following movement challenges:

- Pretend you are a piece of toast coming out of a toaster.
- Show me how a yo-yo moves.
- Can you look like a jack-in-the-box?
- Show me popcorn popping.
- Move up and down like a bouncing ball. A seesaw. An elevator. A balloon inflating and deflating.

Play a bit of "High and Low" for the students, asking them to listen for the sound that gets higher and lower. Once they can identify it, return to the beginning of the song. The children should be sitting. As the music gradually gets higher and higher, the children should raise their arms. Then they lower their arms with the music and rest them where the song provides for it. The pattern follows. If it seems complicated, don't worry; the rising and falling of the music is obvious.

8 counts up; 8 counts down	8 counts up; 4 counts down
8 counts up; 8 counts down	4 counts up; 4 counts down
8-count rest	8-count rest
4 counts up; 4 counts down	2 counts up; 8 counts down; repeat
4 counts up; 4 counts down	2 counts up
8-count rest	
2 counts up; 2 counts down; repeat twice	
8-count rest	

When the children are ready, ask them to crouch low to the ground as you start the song. As the music gradually gets higher and higher, so do the children. Then they descend with the music and rest where the song provides for it. Do it with them at first, later challenging them to do it with the music only as their guide.

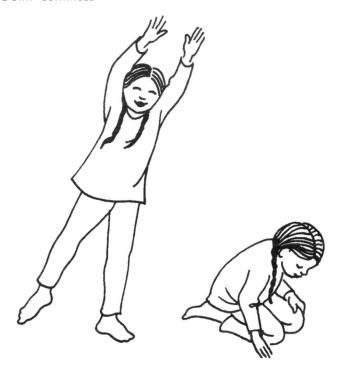

Observation and Evaluation: Does the child demonstrate understanding of the concepts involved? Is the child able to relate to the imagery used? Does the child hear the rising and descending pitch? Does the child respond appropriately?

Adding Equipment: When the children are first doing "High and Low," with arms alone, you can make it a more "colorful" experience by providing them with two scarves apiece—one per hand. Later, you could add a parachute to the whole-body experience. During the eight-count rests, instead of merely waiting, the children can circle the parachute, using whatever traveling skill they prefer (for example, walking, sliding, skipping).

Curriculum Connectors: The levels of high, low, and middle are concepts falling under the headings of both *mathematics* and *art*. Using "High and Low" explores the concept of pitch in *music*. Consideration of the movement of machines such as seesaws, toasters, and elevators constitutes *science*. Listening is one of the four components of *language arts*.

Space Exploration

· ·

♪ "Space Exploration" (Length 2:40)—CD Track 2

Ask the children to get into small, tight body positions on the floor. Once this song begins to play, they begin to uncurl, exploring all the space around them at that low level. You may have to remind them that their personal space includes the area surrounding them, that is, front, back, sides, above, and below. Then, having explored all the space at the lowest level, they *gradually* begin rising (for example, perhaps to one knee, then to both, to a crouch, gradually straightening to a standing position, and perhaps finally onto tiptoe), exploring the space all around them as they rise. Having completed this phase, they can step out of their own personal space into the general space. Lastly, they reverse the whole process until they are back into their small, low body positions.

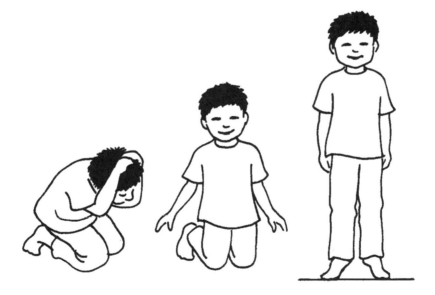

Extending the Activity: Once children have the knack for this, invite them to imagine they are in space capsules that have landed on an unknown planet. When the music starts, they begin by "checking out" all the space immediately surrounding them. They continue the process as outlined above, eventually moving out onto the planet to see what they might find. Finally, they return to their space capsules, where they close themselves in and prepare for the return trip to Earth.

Observation and Evaluation: Does the child understand the concepts of personal and general space? Does the child move successively through the levels? Does the child respect the personal space of others when moving through general space?

Adding Equipment: Starting from and returning to carpet squares, hoops, or poly spots (available from physical education suppliers) can help children with the concept of their own personal space.

Curriculum Connectors: Spatial concepts are a component of *art* and geometry (*mathematics*). You can incorporate *science* by including a discussion of outer space, and *social studies* by talking about the life and role of an astronaut.

Body-Part Relationships

In this activity, the children are going to work with a variety of body parts in relation to other body parts or to the floor. This will require them to think a bit more about the sum of their parts and about the space they occupy.

Ask the children to sit, and then present the following challenges:

- Put an elbow on the floor. Then take it as far away from the floor as possible.
- Stretch a foot far away from you and then bring it back without touching the floor (until it's back in its original position).
- Put a shoulder (the other shoulder; both shoulders) on the floor.
- Touch an elbow to a knee. Then take it as far away from that knee as possible.
- Touch an elbow to a foot.
- Can you touch your shoulder to your foot?
- Touch a wrist to an ankle.
- Come up from the floor with your head leading and the rest of your body following.
- Go back down with an elbow leading the way.
- Come up from the floor with an elbow leading.
- Go back down to the floor with your nose leading the way.
- Come back up with a nose leading.
- Go back down with your chest leading.
- Come back up with your chin leading.

Extending the Activity: A game called Traveling Body Parts will give your students a better idea of the range of their personal space. Ask them to perform the following tasks while standing:

- Make one hand travel far away from the other hand.
- Leaving the first hand (the one that traveled) where it is, bring the other hand to meet it.

- Make the first hand travel far away from the other one, but in a different direction.
- Make one elbow travel far away from the other one.
- Leaving the first elbow where it is, bring the other elbow to meet it.
- Make the first elbow travel far away again, but in a different direction.

Have the children sit and repeat the preceding sequence with knees and feet.

Observation and Evaluation: Does the child have the body and spatial awareness necessary to successfully complete these challenges? Does the child understand the concepts of *apart* and *together*, *far* and *near*?

Adding Equipment: For the initial Traveling Body Parts challenges, holding a scarf or rhythm stick in each hand may make this activity less abstract for some children.

Curriculum Connectors: This body-part experimentation falls under the heading of *science* for young children. Because it explores personal space and levels, it involves *art* concepts as well. Together, apart, far, and near are important positional concepts in both art and *mathematics*.

Exploring Body and Spatial Directions

Ask the children to each find their own personal space and to remember where that space is. Then stand in the center of the room where everyone can see you, acting as a point of reference, and present the following challenges:

- Walk to me, turn, and go back to your own space.
- Walk forward to me, but return to your space sideways.
- Walk sideways to me, and return to your space backward.
- Walk backward to me, and return to your space in a forward direction.

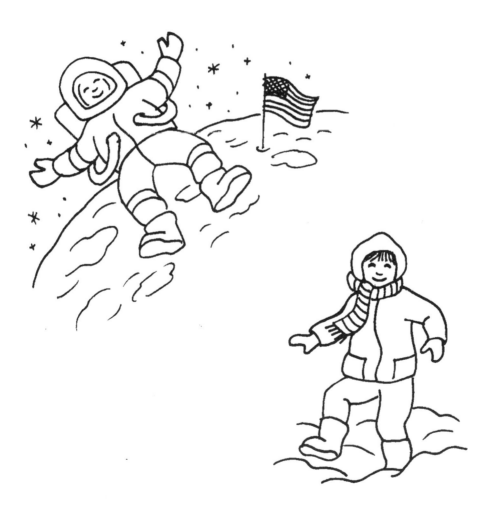

Extending the Activity: You can further challenge children to approach and retreat from you in the following ways:

- in a straight path
- from one side; from the other side
- from the back
- in a curving path; a zigzagging one

Ask the children to really use their imaginations by challenging them to approach and retreat from you as though in the following situations:

- on slippery ice
- on hot sand that is burning their feet
- in deep snow
- in sticky mud
- on the moon and weightless
- through thick fog
- in a jungle with thick growth
- on a busy, crowded sidewalk

Observation and Evaluation: Does the child demonstrate the ability to move in the directions cited? Can the child move without interfering with the movement of others? Does the child identify with the imagery used?

Adding Equipment: Using hoops, carpet squares, or poly spots can help children identify and remember their own personal spaces.

Curriculum Connectors: Direction and space are components of *art*. Directionality is also critical to reading and writing (*language arts*). And the self-expression promoted through the extension activity brings in *social studies*.

Making Shapes

Shape is a movement element that is fun to explore in your own personal space. Making sure the children have enough room to respond without touching one another, ask them the following:

- How round can you be?
- How flat can you be? Wide? Narrow? Long? Short? Crooked? Straight?
- Make your body look like a table. A chair.
- Show me you can look like a ball. A pencil with a point at the end. A flower. A teapot. A rug.

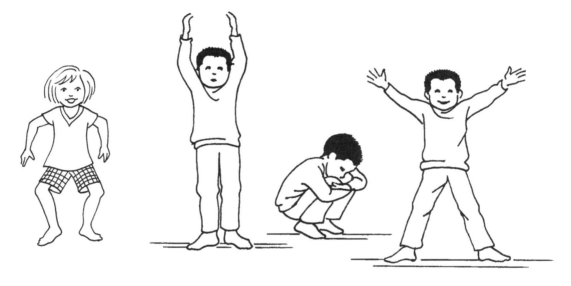

Extending the Activity: Show the children construction paper cutouts of different shapes (for example, squares, triangles, circles, rectangles), or point out items in the room (for example, a desk, a chair, the blackboard, a jacket). Then ask your students to imitate these shapes, one at a time, with their bodies.

A game called Changing Shapes is more challenging still. With the children each in their own personal space, choose three different shapes (for example, high, low, and wide), and assign an order to them (for example, the first shape is high, the second is low, and the third is wide). Now instruct the children to move slowly from the first to the second to the third and then back to the first, with a pause as each shape is attained. Next have them move from one shape to another continuously, without any pauses. Other possibilities include the following:

- moving quickly from one shape to another
- moving slowly from the first to the second and then quickly to the third and back to the first, and so on
- moving strongly, as though against resistance; then lightly

Observation and Evaluation: Does the child understand the concept of shape? Is the child able to replicate shapes appropriately?

Adding Equipment: The children will have great fun trying these shapes from inside Body Sox (a stretchy fabric available from physical education suppliers)! If possible, take pictures of their shapes and let them see what they have created.

Curriculum Connectors: Shape is integral to both *art* and *mathematics*. Being able to physically replicate what the eyes see is a skill necessary in writing (*language arts*).

Directing Traffic

Using prearranged hand signals for *forward, backward, move right, move left, turn,* and *walk in place*, direct the children in their movement as though you are directing traffic. Until the children have had a lot of experience with this, they should simply use the locomotor skill of walking for the activity. (*Note:* All of the children must be facing the same direction— toward you—in order for this to work.)

Extending the Activity: Play a game of Coming and Going. Using a hand clap or a drum, beat out a moderate walking tempo. The children walk forward at this tempo until you call out a number. The children must then take that number of steps backward *at the same tempo,* and then go forward again. Some suggestions for making this activity successful include the following:

- Keep a steady tempo that does not speed up or slow down.
- You may want to repeat each number twice in a row so the children have two chances to succeed.
- Because of the tempo, even numbers may be easier for the children at first.
- Similarly, higher numbers (four and above) may prove easier at first.
- The children should be as spread out as possible to reduce the possibility of collision.

Observation and Evaluation: Is the child able to follow your visual directions? Is the child taking the correct number of steps? Is the child able to maintain a constant tempo?

Adding Equipment: Having each child simultaneously beat a hand drum or rhythm sticks during the extension activity can add another two senses, auditory and kinesthetic, to the experience and help make it more challenging and fun!

Curriculum Connectors: Direction is a component of *art*, while tempo is an element of *music*. Counting, of course, is a *mathematics* skill.

Moving Slow/Moving Fast

♪ **"Moving Slow/Moving Fast" (Length 2:44)—CD Track 3**

Play this song, consisting of slow sections (A) and fast sections (B), suggesting the children move in the following ways to each. The form of the song is ABAB.

Slow music	**Fast Music**
tiptoeing	fast walking
floating weightlessly	taking tiny steps
taking soft, giant steps	shaking all over
swaying	jumping lightly

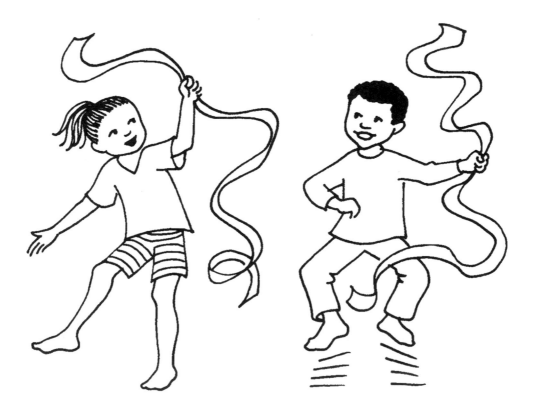

Extending the Activity: Once the children can easily recognize the difference in tempo, encourage them to find their own ways of moving to the slow and fast music. Does it make them feel like moving in different ways?

When children are familiar with the contrast between fast and slow, ask them to pretend to be things that are either fast or slow. You may choose to complete one category before moving to the other, or you can alternate between the two categories. Generally, young children will find it easier to perform fast movements.

Fast	Slow
a fire engine	a turtle
a jet plane	the hands of a clock
an arrow	a snail
the wind	a train just starting up
a cheetah	the sun rising
a spaceship	a snowman melting

Observation and Evaluation: Can the child recognize the difference between the slow and fast tempos? Do the child's movements show a marked difference between slow and fast? Does the child identify with the imagery used?

Adding Equipment: Giving the children a prop to move, such as a scarf, streamer, or ribbon stick, can help alleviate any self-consciousness and also allows them to see the difference between slow and fast movements.

Curriculum Connectors: This song explores the concept of tempo in *music* and the movement element of time, which falls under the heading of *mathematics* for young children. The original activity also involved adjectives and adverbs (*language arts*).

Slow-Motion Moving

♪ **"Slow-Motion Moving" (Length 2:16)—CD Track 4**

Choose different locomotor and nonlocomotor skills, and ask the children to perform them in slow motion, as though in a movie with the film slowed down, to the accompaniment of "Slow-Motion Moving." Possible skills include walking, running, swinging arms, and swaying.

Extending the Activity: When your students are developmentally ready, ask them to create a short sequence of movements—perhaps as though they were participating in a sport—and, after practicing it to achieve consistency, have them perform it in slow motion, as though in instant replay.

Observation and Evaluation: Does the child understand the concept of slow motion? Does the child demonstrate the control necessary to move slowly?

Adding Equipment: For the activity extension, you could make a piece of sports equipment—for example, a tennis racket, baseball bat, golf club, or some kind of ball—available to each child. If a ball is used, the sequence should not involve actually throwing it.

Curriculum Connectors: These activities involve the element of tempo in *music* and time in movement, which falls under the heading of *mathematics*.

Exploring Accelerando and Ritardando

. . . .

♪ **"Getting Fast/Getting Slow" (Length 2:25)—CD Track 5**

Before beginning, explain the terms *accelerando* (ah-che-luh-RAHN-doh) and *ritardando* (rih-tar-DAHN-doh) to your students. *Accelerando* is the term used for music or movement that gradually increases in tempo. *Ritardando* is the opposite—gradually slowing.

In this follow-the-leader activity, you should have the children form a line behind you and then perform movements that accelerate. Next, when you reach a maximum tempo, gradually slow down. Walking is the simplest activity to perform, but you might also use jogging, tiptoeing, hopping, or jumping.

Extending the Activity: "Getting Fast/Getting Slow" is a musical example of accelerando and ritardando. The form of the song is ABAB, with A demonstrating accelerando and B ritardando.

Using a walk, lead the children around the room, increasing and decreasing your speed with the tempo of the music. If you find the children are having difficulty with this or are becoming restless, feel free to call it quits after AB.

Once children have the knack for this, challenge them to perform the activity in pairs, shadowing one another. The lead partner matches the tempo of the music and the following partner matches the lead partner's movements. After AB, partners switch roles.

To explore ritardando only, talk to the children about wind-up toys and how they move, both when they have been newly wound and when they are winding down. Then ask the children to choose the wind-up toys they would like to be (possibilities include dolls, dogs, monkeys, clowns, or another toy), and "wind them up" as a whole or individually, if your group is small enough.

The children should begin by moving quickly and then eventually begin to get slower. When completely wound down, they should either come to a stop or topple to the floor.

Observation and Evaluation: Is the child able to imitate your (or a partner's) movements?

Does the child demonstrate the control required to gradually speed up and slow down? Does the child successfully move in a group or with a partner?

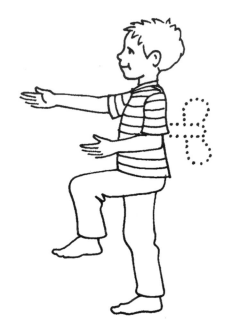

Curriculum Connectors: These activities offer experiences with two elements of *music*, which go hand in hand with the movement element of time (a component of *mathematics*). The activities also require group and partner cooperation, incorporating *social studies*.

Soft and Loud

♪ "Moving Softly/Moving Loudly" (Length 2:47)—CD Track 6

♪ "Getting Louder/Getting Softer" (Length 2:31)—CD Track 7

The form of "Moving Softly/Moving Loudly" is ABAB, with A being the soft section. Offer the following suggestions to the children, one at a time, as they move to the music.

Soft	Loud
tiptoeing	stamping feet
moving arms gently	punching toward the
patting the floor	sky
swaying gently	pounding the floor
	rocking forcefully

Extending the Activity: Once children can distinguish between the soft and loud music, challenge them to move in any way they like to the soft and loud sections. Can they find new ways to move?

The next step is to explain the terms *crescendo* (kruh-SHEN-doh) and *decrescendo* (day-kruh-SHEN-doh) the children. Both musical terms refer to the volume of a musical passage. When there is a crescendo, the volume gradually gets louder. A decrescendo is just the opposite. The volume gradually gets softer. Play "Getting Louder/Getting Softer," the form of which is ABAB, with A demonstrating crescendo and B decrescendo.

You can begin by tiptoeing around the room with the children, either in a scattered form or with them in a line behind you, gradually increasing the weight of your steps as the music grows louder. By the time the volume is at its loudest, you should be stamping your feet. The music then begins to grow softer, as should your steps, until you are tiptoeing once again. The sequence is then repeated.

Once children are familiar with this concept, they can perform the activity in pairs, one shadowing another. After a while, partners reverse roles.

Observation and Evaluation: Can the child distinguish between soft and loud? Does the child demonstrate movements appropriate to soft and loud music? Does the child demonstrate the understanding and control necessary to gradually increase and decrease the force of the movement?

Adding Equipment: How might a prop, like a scarf, streamer, or ribbon stick, move to the soft and loud music?

Curriculum Connectors: This activity involves the concept of volume (*music*) and the movement element of force, which is a quantitative concept falling under the heading of *mathematics*. The cooperative nature of the partner activity constitutes *social studies*.

Robots and Astronauts

. . . .

♪ **"Robots and Astronauts" (Length 3:19)—CD Track 8**

Play this song, the form of which is ABAB. During A, the children pretend to move like robots (stiffly and mechanically). During B, they pretend to float in space like weightless astronauts.

Extending the Activity: With repetitions of this activity, you can make it a bit more challenging by issuing follow-up questions to vary the children's responses. For example, you might ask the following:

- Is there some way those robots might use their heads as they move?
- Is there another direction (pathway) the robots might move in?
- Can the astronauts float in different directions?
- Is there another shape the astronauts might float in?

Observation and Evaluation: This is an exercise in both flow (bound and free) and force. Does the child differentiate between the bound movement of the robot and the free movement of the astronaut? Does the child exhibit a difference in muscle tension from one to the other?

Curriculum Connectors: This song exhibits both form and a contrast between staccato (short, separated notes) and legato (longer, smooth-flowing notes) in *music*. Focusing on muscle tension offers an experience in *science*.

Staccato/Legato

· ·

♪ **"Staccato/Legato" (Length 3:13)—CD Track 9**

This song offers experience with the musical elements of *staccato* and *legato* and the movement element of flow. Explain the two musical terms to the children. *Staccato* (stuh-CAH-toh) is short and separated notes and tends to inspire movement using a bound flow. *Legato* (lih-GAH-toh) is smooth and can be likened to free flow.

The form of the song is ABAB, with A representing staccato and B legato. Offer the following suggestions for movement:

Staccato	Legato
a robot moving	a butterfly floating
tiptoeing	ice skating
a stalking cat	an eagle soaring
a battery-operated toy	a weightless astronaut

Extending the Activity: When repeating this activity, ask the children to simply show you how these two kinds of music make them feel like moving. You might also ask them to experiment with moving in the *opposite* way to each kind of music. Does it work?

Observation and Evaluation: Can the child differentiate between staccato and legato? Does the child move appropriately to each?

Adding Equipment: Make a variety of props available to the children, allowing them to choose which props work best for each section of the music. Possible props include streamers, ribbon sticks, maracas, hand drums, scarves, rhythm sticks, wooden blocks, and hoops.

Curriculum Connectors: Staccato and legato fall under the broader category of articulation in *music*. Listening is one of the four components of *language arts*.

Exploring Opposites

Discuss the meaning of *opposites* with the children, and then explain that you are going to give them an instruction to do something. They will first respond by doing what you asked, but then they will do the opposite—without being told what the opposite is.

Possible challenges include the following:

- Make yourself very tall.
- Show me how flat you can be.
- Show me tiny steps.
- Move as though you were very sad.
- Move as lightly as a feather.
- Show me how slowly you can move.
- Let me see a wide shape.
- Show me a frowning face.

Extending the Activity: When the students are comfortable with this concept, ask them to work with a partner. One partner will demonstrate a movement or shape, with the second partner demonstrating the opposite. The second partner begins the next set.

Observation and Evaluation: Does the child understand the concept of opposites? Does the child appropriately demonstrate opposites?

Curriculum Connectors: The concept of opposites is a part of *language arts*, while the cooperative nature of the extension activity falls under the heading of *social studies*.

Bending and Stretching

Invite the children to experiment with bending and stretching a variety of body parts in a variety of directions. How many body parts can be bent and stretched—and in how many ways? Remind them to be gentle!

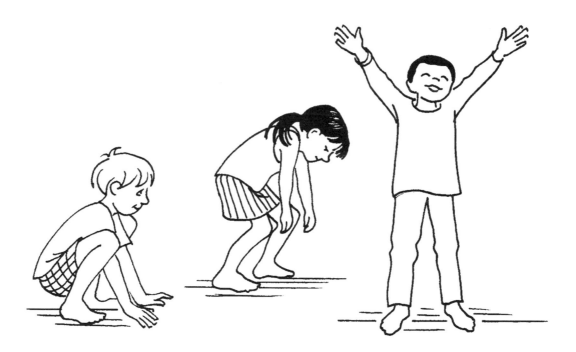

Extending the Activity: Here we use imagery to explore the nonlocomotor skills of bending and stretching. Feel free to add some of your own ideas, but remember that the children must be able to relate to the images you choose.

Have the children do the following:

- Stretch as though picking fruit from a tall tree.
- Flop like a rag doll.
- Stretch as though waking up and yawning first thing in the morning.
- Bend as though to tie shoes.
- Stretch to put something on a high shelf.

- Bend to pat a dog; an even smaller dog, or a cat.
- Stretch to shoot a basketball through a hoop.
- Bend to pick up a coin from the floor.
- Stretch as though climbing a ladder.
- Bend to pick vegetables or flowers from a garden.

Observation and Evaluation: Does the child differentiate between bending and stretching? Does the child identify with the imagery involved?

Curriculum Connectors: The concepts of up, down, high, and low fall under the headings of both *mathematics* and *art* (spatial relationships).

Exploring Bending and Stretching

Bending and stretching are the simplest of the nonlocomotor skills to perform, and they have already been introduced to the children. However, the skills are made more challenging here because the students are being asked to bend or stretch more than one body part at a time.

Pose the following challenges:

- Show me you can stretch one arm high and the other low (one toward the ceiling and the other toward the floor).
- Bend one arm while stretching the other high. Low. To the side.
- Reach both arms to the right (one side). To the left (the other side).
- Reach one arm to the side and the other toward the ceiling.
- On hands and knees, stretch one leg behind you and one arm forward.
- Lying on your back, stretch one leg and bend the other.
- Stretch one leg long and the other toward the ceiling.

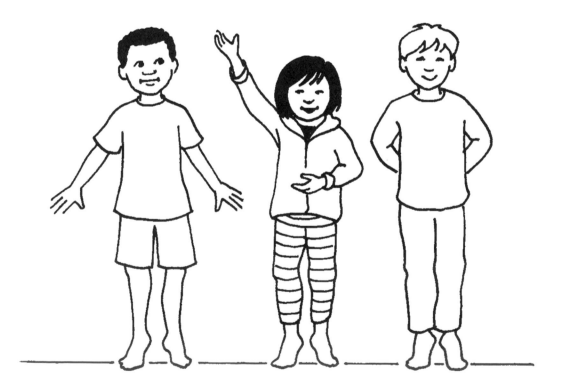

Extending the Activity: Invite the children to discover how many other body parts can be both bent *and* stretched? Which parts can do only one or the other?

Observation and Evaluation: Does the child understand the concepts of bending and stretching? Is the child able to bend and stretch in opposition? Does the child understand the directions?

Adding Equipment: Giving the children a pencil and paper to record their findings can spark interest in the extended activity and encourage more serious probing.

Curriculum Connectors: Exploring the capabilities and limitations of body parts constitutes *science*, while the spatial concepts of high, low, up, down, forward, and backward fall under the headings of both *mathematics* and *art*.

Let's Shake

 "Shake It High/Shake It Low" (Length 2:58)—CD Track 10

With this exercise, children will discover they can shake various body parts, as well as the whole body, and at different levels in space. Issue the following challenges:

- Shake your whole body.
- Sit and shake just one hand; the other; both together.
- Shake your hands in front of you; to either side; up high; down low.
- Find another part of your body to shake; another.
- Kneeling, how many parts of your body can you find to shake?
- Lie on your back and shake one part; another; your whole body.
- Is it easier or harder to shake while lying on your tummy?

Extending the Activity: Discuss the meaning of the words *shaking, wiggling,* and *vibrating* with the children and ask them to show you they can do the following:

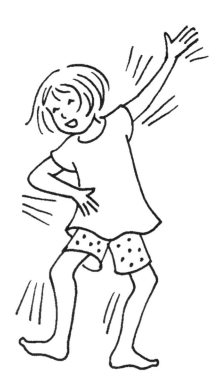

- move like a snake
- move like soup when the bowl is shaken
- shake and vibrate like a baby's rattle
- quiver like a leaf in the wind
- shiver as though very, very cold
- shake like a battery-powered toothbrush

The song "Shake It High/Shake It Low" provides some additional experience with the skill of shaking, as well as the three levels in space and the isolation of body parts. When the chorus calls for shaking "in the middle," it refers to shaking the body or part at the middle level (standing). Here are the lyrics:

Shaking is a way to have some fun,
So let's shake our bodies, everyone!
Your head sits at the top of you.
Believe it or not, it can shake too!
There are many ways to shake a hand,
But up in the air will be just grand!
To "shake a leg" can mean to hurry,
But quick or slow, no need to worry!

It can be fun to shake your bottom,
So shake those hips—that's why you've
  got 'em!
Shoulders are a little bit harder,
But you can try, just for a starter!
Chorus: *Show me you can shake it high.*
Show me you can shake it low.
Shake it in the middle.
And away we go!

Observation and Evaluation: Does the child understand the concept of shaking? Is the child able to shake a variety of body parts? Does the child relate to the imagery involved? Does the child demonstrate understanding of the three levels in space? (*Note:* Developmentally, it is still too soon to expect the children to be able to isolate individual body parts to the extent that they move *only* that part. Most likely, if a child is shaking his or her head, most of the rest of the body is also shaking!)

Adding Equipment: You might want to have maracas handy—either for demonstration purposes or to hand out to the children to add to the fun of shaking.

Curriculum Connectors: Body-part identification and experimenting with the capabilities and limitations of body parts qualifies as *science* for young children. Using the song adds both *music* and *language arts.*

Let's Sway

♪ **"Swaying Song" (Length 2:02)—CD Track 11**

Demonstrate swaying to the children, explaining that a *sway* transfers weight from one part of the body to another in an easy, relaxed motion. Then ask them to try swaying from side to side and back and forth.

Next, add some imagery to the activity by asking them to sway like the following things:

- flowers in the breeze
- rocking horses (or rocking chairs)
- bells ringing
- windshield wipers

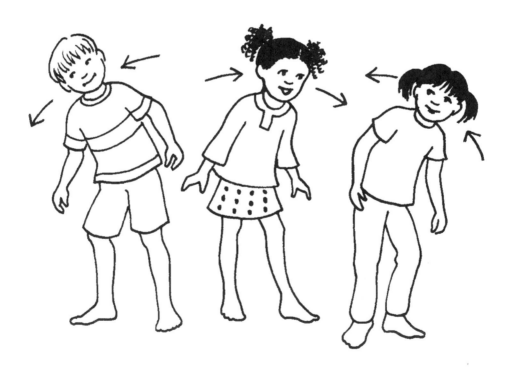

Extending the Activity: When the children are ready to perform the sway to the accompaniment of music, ask them to stand in a circle, and then put on the "Swaying Song." Ask the children to sway in the following ways:

- without touching one another
- holding hands
- with arms on one another's shoulders
- with arms around one another's waists

Eventually, while in the latter position, challenge them to increase the sway just a bit so one foot is coming slightly off the floor (if they are swaying to the right, the left foot will lift, and vice versa).

Observation and Evaluation: Does the child properly execute a sway—alone and with others? Does the child demonstrate the balance and recovery required of swaying until one foot lifts off the floor?

Adding Equipment: When moving individually, swaying a ribbon stick or streamer simultaneously can help the child correctly perform a sway by imitating the look and feel of the prop.

Curriculum Connectors: Using the song incorporates *music*. Balance and recovery are components of *science*. The extension activity requires cooperation, which falls under the heading of *social studies*.

Let's Sit

Although sitting may be a skill primary-grade students have long since mastered, it can still be a challenging activity when explored at a variety of levels, especially with the additional movement elements of time and force. Explain this to the children, and then present the following challenges:

- Sit from a standing position, using your hands to let you down.
- Do it again, only this time without using your hands.
- Sit down very slowly.
- Sit with a thump.
- Sit with the weight on your right (left) thigh.

Extending the Activity: Additional challenges might include the following:

- From a kneeling position, sit down gently.
- From a kneeling position, sit down with a thump.
- From a kneeling position, sit with the weight on your right (left) thigh.
- Sit up from a lying position.
- Show me how slowly you can sit up from a lying position.

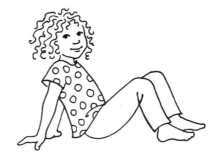

Observation and Evaluation: Does the child demonstrate the control necessary to perform these tasks? Does the child understand what is expected?

Adding Equipment: Performing these tasks within a hoop or on a poly spot can make them more visual and colorful, thereby making them more fun.

Curriculum Connectors: This is an exploration of the levels in space, which can be linked to *art* and *mathematics*.

Let's Turn

Children love to turn themselves around and make themselves dizzy. In this activity, however, they will be introduced to the nonlocomotor skill of turning as a *controlled* movement—a rotation of the body around an axis that can occur in a great variety of ways.

Pose the following questions and challenges:

- Turn yourself around to the right (one way). To the left (the other way).
- Show me you can turn yourself around very, very slowly.
- Turn while being as tall (small) as you can.
- Show me you can turn while on your knees. On one knee.
- Turn while sitting on your bottom.
- Turn on just one foot.
- Jump and turn at the same time.
- Can you turn in the air?

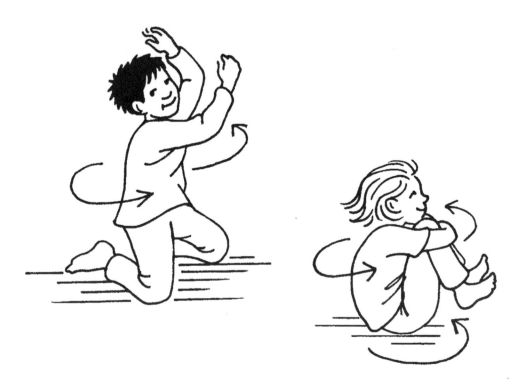

Extending the Activity: Additional challenges include the following:

- Turn like an airplane would turn as it comes in for a landing.
- Hop and turn at the same time.
- Turn being as round (crooked) as you can be.
- Turn quickly and very gradually slow down.
- Turn slowly one way and even slower the other way.
- Turn quickly one way and even quicker the other way.
- Turn in one direction for eight counts. ("Which way do you end up facing?")
- Turn in the other direction for four counts and end facing front.

Observation and Evaluation: A turn is a partial or complete rotation of the body around an axis, causing shift in weight placement. Does the child display an ability to correctly execute half and full turns with control and in a variety of ways?

Adding Equipment: Executing turns while standing inside a hoop can help children understand this is a nonlocomotor skill. It is also fun to turn while holding a streamer or ribbon stick.

Curriculum Connectors: The concept of rotation around an axis is simple *science*, as is the balance required to turn in a controlled manner.

Let's Twist

 "Twisting" (Length 2:02)—CD Track 12

Unlike a turn, which rotates the whole body, a twist rotates a *part* of the body around an axis. It is perhaps through imagery that early elementary children can best relate to the nonlocomotor skill of twisting. With that in mind, ask them to twist in these ways:

- like the inside of a washing machine
- like a screwdriver when someone is using it
- like a wet dishrag being wrung
- as though wiping their bottoms with towels
- as though digging a little hole in the sand with a foot
- as though wiping with a towel and digging a little hole in the sand with a foot at the same time

Extending the Activity: Repeat the above activities, accompanying the movement with the song "Twisting." Also challenge children to discover how many body parts, besides the trunk, can twist. Possibilities include arms, legs, and neck, with wrists, ankles, shoulders, and hips able to twist to a lesser extent.

Observation and Evaluation: Does the child identify with the imagery used? Does the child differentiate between a twist and a turn?

Curriculum Connectors: Using the song incorporates *music*, while experimentation with the capabilities and limitations of body parts involves *science*.

Let's Walk

 "Walking Along" (Length 1:41)—CD Track 13

This activity provides an excellent opportunity for you to observe the children's strengths and weaknesses with regard to posture and alignment, weight distribution, and use of body parts—while the children simply have fun walking. Observing closely, have the children walk in the following ways:

- freely (while being straight and tall)
- in place ("Can you make your knees go higher? Can you do it faster?")
- forward ("Can you do it slower?")
- on tiptoe ("Can you make yourself even taller?")
- on heels (briefly)
- very slowly; very quickly
- with tiny steps; with giant steps
- very lightly; very strongly
- walk-walk-stop; repeat

Extending the Activity: When the children are ready, challenge them to walk in sideways and backward directions (space), reminding them to be even more careful when moving among their classmates. To increase the challenge, combine two movement elements, offering challenges like the following:

- Walk forward on your heels (*space* and *shape*).
- Walk backward on tiptoe.
- Walk sideways while making your body very small.
- Walk slowly in a curving pathway (*time* and *space*).
- Walk quickly in a zigzagging pathway.
- Walk as quickly and lightly as you can (*time* and *force*).

To incorporate rhythm, accompany any of the above activities with the "Walking Along" song. Don't worry if the children do not move "at one" with the beat of the music; it will all come in good time.

Incorporate imagery into the exploration of this locomotor skill by asking the children to walk like they are the following:

- really mad; sad; tired; proud; scared
- looking for the towel with soap in your eyes
- in a parade
- on hot sand that is burning your feet
- trying to get through sticky mud; deep snow; an overgrown jungle
- on slippery ice
- on a crowded city sidewalk

Observation and Evaluation: Does the child demonstrate proper posture and alignment, with weight distributed evenly over all five toes and the heel of the foot? Does the child respond to the imagery used?

Adding Equipment: Play "Walking Along," inviting the children to accompany the song with rhythm instruments. Challenge them to roll a hoop, to balance a beanbag on different body parts, or circle a ribbon stick overhead or to one side while walking.

Curriculum Connectors: By accompanying the activity with "Walking Along," you are incorporating *music*. Because self-discovery, including the exploration of emotions, is the first step in *social studies* for young children, using the imagery suggested incorporates that content area.

Let's Run

 "The Track Meet" (Length 1:21)—CD Track 14

Challenge the children to run in the following ways:

- in place ("Can you make your knees go higher? Can you go faster? Slower?")
- forward; backward
- in a circle
- making a lot of noise with the feet
- very lightly, with tiny steps
- starting and stopping on signal

Extending the Activity: Add imagery to the locomotor skill of running. Stressing realism, ask the children to run as though they are doing the following:

- carrying a football in the big game
- trying to catch a bus
- crossing very hot sand at the beach
- being chased by somebody
- dribbling a basketball down the court
- finishing a long, exhausting race
- flying a kite
- carrying very heavy loads on their backs

You can accompany all of these activities and motions with "The Track Meet" to provide the children with musical motivation and an audible running rhythm. Maybe the children would like to imagine they are running in the Olympics!

Observation and Evaluation: Does the child run with the proper body alignment, with the body's weight transferred from the ball and toes of one foot to the ball and toes of the other? Is the body inclined slightly forward, with the arms bent and swinging in opposition to the legs? Does the child identify with the imagery involved?

Curriculum Connectors: Use of the song incorporates *music*, while a discussion of the Olympics and the self-expression in the extension activity can embrace *social studies*.

Let's Jump

A jump propels the body upward from a takeoff on two feet. The toes, which are the last to leave the ground (heel-ball-toe), are the first to reach it upon landing, with landings occurring toe-ball-heel and with both knees bent. Ask the children to experiment with jumping in the following ways:

- in place ("Show me you can you do it with your feet barely coming off the floor. With your feet coming way off. Can you make your knees go higher? Show me you can jump fast. Jump being as tall as you can. As small.")
- forward ("To that point over there; in a circle; very slowly.")
- backward ("Making a lot of noise with your feet. Very lightly, as though jumping on eggs and you don't want to break them.")

Extending the Activity: Add some imagery to the exercise, asking the children to jump in these ways:

- as though they are bouncing balls (some high, some low)
- pretending to reach for something above them
- as though startled by a loud noise
- as though angry (having a tantrum)
- with joy

Invite the children to explore jumping in these more challenging ways:

- with feet together; apart
- with feet alternately apart and together
- landing with one foot forward and the other back
- clicking heels together while in the air
- with arms held still by their sides
- with arms folded across chest
- with arms extended forward; upward; to the sides
- with hands on hips

- with hands clasped behind the back
- with hands clapping

Observation and Evaluation: Is the child achieving elevation by pushing off from the toes? Does the child land with knees bent and heels coming all the way down to the floor? Does the child maintain a correct posture while jumping and landing?

Curriculum Connectors: Incorporate *science* by discussing (simply) the concept of gravity. In other words, why don't we stay up in the air when we jump? The self-expression in the extension activity brings in *social studies*.

Let's Leap

Demonstrate a leap to your students, explaining that it is similar to a run, except that the knee and ankle action is greater. Early elementary children may be able to relate best to this locomotor skill through imagery. For example, you can ask them to pretend to leap in the following ways:

- over a puddle
- over a tall building (like a superhero)
- like a deer over fallen trees in the forest
- over a hurdle in the Olympics

Extending the Activity: Children will first lead with the preferred leg. Be sure to encourage them to try leaping with the nonpreferred leg leading as well.

After the children have had ample experience with leaping, challenge them to combine leaping with running. Ask them to do these movements:

- perform several leaps in a row without stops in between
- run several steps then leap; repeat
- run, leap; run, leap; and so on
- run, run, leap; run, run, leap; and so on

Observation and Evaluation: Following takeoff, does the child lead with the knee and then extend it as the foot reaches forward to land? Does the back leg extend to the rear while the child is in the air? Does the child raise the arms to assist with elevation?

Adding Equipment: Some children relate better to leaping when it is performed over a prop, like a rope held just an inch or two off the floor. Again, be sure they practice leading with both legs. To challenge all children at their own skill levels, have two children hold the rope at a slant, with one end very near the floor and the other several inches above it. Students can choose to jump over the rope at the point at which they feel most comfortable.

Curriculum Connectors: To incorporate *science*, discuss the concept of gravity with the children, reminding them it is the reason they don't stay in the air when they leap.

Let's Gallop

♪ **"Giddy-Up" (Length 1:39)—CD Track 15**

A gallop is a locomotor skill unlike the walk and the run in that it is performed with an uneven rhythm. It is a combination of a walk and a leap in which one foot leads and the other plays catch-up.

Introduce the children to the gallop, keeping in mind that it is best learned by imitation or by holding hands and moving with someone who knows how to gallop. For those not ready to perform an actual gallop, you can simply suggest moving "like a horse."

Extending the Activity: Play "Giddy-Up" and have the children "saddle up and ride." If space is a problem, you may want to have them gallop in a circle or in rounds (one small group at a time). The song offers brief rest periods to prepare the next group to begin, or for "stopping at a watering hole."

Once children have mastered leading with the preferred foot, challenge them to lead with the other foot.

Challenge students to gallop in curving and zigzagging pathways, lightly and strongly, slowly and quickly, and changing directions often.

Observation and Evaluation: Does the child consistently lead with one foot, with the other following (but not passing)? Is the child's galloping rhythm uneven? Can the child lead with the nonpreferred foot?

Adding Equipment: Provide children with sets of rhythm sticks so they can accompany their movements with an audible rhythm.

Curriculum Connectors: A discussion of how horses move can bring a bit of *science* to this activity, which also offers experience with *music* and rhythm (also central to *language arts*).

Let's Hop

A hop is a movement that propels the body upward from a takeoff on *one* foot. The landing is then made on the same foot, toe-ball-heel, with the knee bent. The free leg does not come in contact with the ground.

Demonstrate a hop to the children, and then ask them to show you hopping. You may find that some have more success hopping in place, whereas others find it easier to hop around the room. If some children have trouble maintaining balance, you might pair them up and ask them to hold hands, lift their outside legs, and hop together.

Extending the Activity: Children will hop first on the preferred foot. Once they have had ample experience with that, encourage them to try hopping on the nonpreferred foot. The next step is to invite them to hop around the room, changing feet often.

Observation and Evaluation: Is the child able to maintain balance? Does the child land with a bent knee, with the heel coming all the way to the floor? Can the child hop on both the preferred and non-preferred foot?

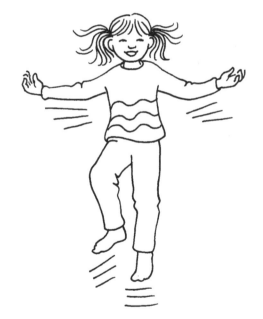

Adding Equipment: Place one hoop per child on the floor, challenging the children to hop in and out, all the way around it. Also, place carpet squares or poly spots in a row on the floor, inviting the children to hop from one to the next. This can make hopping more fun for the children.

Curriculum Connectors: A discussion of gravity, the reason we can't stay in the air when we hop, can link this activity to *science*, as does the concept of balance.

Let's Slide

A slide resembles a gallop in that one foot leads and the other plays catch-up in an uneven rhythm. In a slide, however, the movement is to the side rather than forward. (Facing forward, with feet together, the child slides one leg out to the side and then, with the weight primarily on that leg, slides the second leg in, so that the feet are once again together. The action, therefore, is step-close, step-close.) Demonstrate the slide to the children and then have them practice it to both sides.

Extending the Activity: When the children are ready, introduce some variations to the slide, remembering to have them slide to both the left and right side. For example, ask them if they can slide in these ways:

- quickly; slowly
- lightly; heavily
- in a circle
- with their arms out to the sides; above their heads

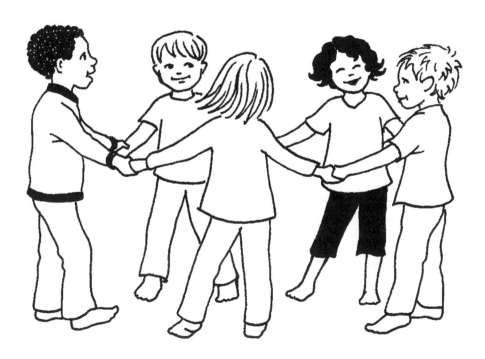

Next, challenge them to slide in both directions with a partner, making at least one physical contact (holding hands, hands on shoulders, and so on). Finally, challenge the whole class to perform the movement in a circle, holding hands. Ask them to begin with a gallop around the circle first, then to turn to face the center of the circle, and to slide in unison around the circle. Can they move sideways rhythmically to the accompaniment of your hands clapping? Can they lead with either foot, circling in both directions? Can they circle first in one direction (for example, to eight counts) and then the other, changing directions smoothly?

Observation and Evaluation: Is the child able to face one direction and move in another? Does the child perform the slide with an uneven rhythm? Can the child slide in both directions?

Adding Equipment: Sliding is a locomotor skill commonly used to move a parachute in a circle. You might also want to beat out the correct rhythm on a hand drum to add another sense to the experience, and especially to assist the auditory learners.

Curriculum Connectors: Accompanying the children's movements with a drum places greater emphasis on the rhythm, which is an element of both *music* and *language arts*. Sliding with partners and as a group, because it is a cooperative activity, offers an experience in *social studies*.

Let's Skip

♪ "Skipping Song" (Length 1:09)—CD Track 16

A skip is actually a combination of two locomotor skills—a step and a hop. Like the gallop, a skip consists of an uneven rhythm. With more emphasis placed on the step than the hop, the overall effect is that of a light and skimming motion during which the feet only momentarily lose contact with the ground.

If necessary, introduce skipping to the children, explaining that the skip is a combination of a step and a hop. There are many ways to teach skipping, but you will have to find a method that works with your particular group. Some children have learned to skip by pretending the floor was very hot and that as soon as they stepped on it with one foot they would want to hop right back off it (and then repeat with the other foot). Some children may learn by imitation and others by holding hands and skipping with someone who knows how. This latter method is particularly effective for children who can skip on one side and not the other (have them hold hands on the side on which they cannot skip).

For those children who can already perform this locomotor skill, play "Skipping Song" and ask the children to accompany it with skipping. Some children may find the rhythm of the music helps them.

Extending the Activity: Once the children are skipping successfully, provide some variety by suggesting they skip in circles, as lightly as possible, quickly, and in curving and zigzagging paths. Can they skip backward? The next challenge is to invite them to skip with partners, making at least one physical contact (holding hands, hands on shoulders, and so on).

Observation and Evaluation: Is the child able to skip on both sides of the body? Does the child demonstrate the appropriate rhythm? Does the child use arms in opposition to the legs? Does the child maintain the proper posture?

Adding Equipment: Some children are aided in their quest to skip with vinyl cutout feet placed in a path on the floor.

Curriculum Connectors: In addition to the focus on rhythm, using the song provides experience with *music*, as does the focus on rhythm, which is also central to *language arts*.

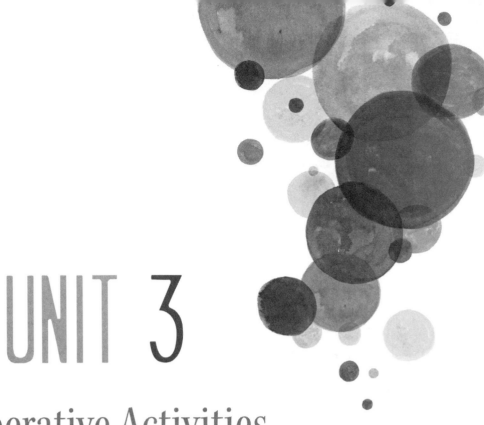

UNIT 3

Cooperative Activities

The activities in this unit serve three purposes: (1) They offer students opportunities to work cooperatively with partners and in small and large groups. (2) They provide greater challenge, beyond what the children experience in unit 2. (3) These activities can physically and emotionally prepare the students to successfully work together in the educational gymnastics and rhythm and dance activities in units 4 and 5 requiring participation in pairs or groups.

Bridges and Tunnels

The children pair up, and one partner forms a bridge or tunnel, which the other child goes over or under. That child then forms a bridge that is different from her or his partner's, and the process continues.

The children should be given enough time to experiment and explore, but not so much time that they become bored with this challenge.

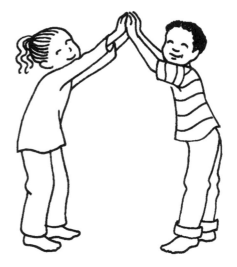

Extending the Activity: Challenge *trios* of children to form two-person bridges and tunnels, which the third student goes over or under. Children take turns in each role, trying to find as many possible solutions to the challenge as they can.

Observation and Evaluation: Does the child work cooperatively with others? Is the child able to find a variety of solutions to each challenge?

Adding Equipment: Children can enhance their responses with the aid of hoops or ropes. However, their bodies must still be part of the solution.

Curriculum Connectors: A discussion about the role bridges and tunnels play in transportation can add an element of *social studies* over and above the cooperative aspect. These activities are also an exploration of shape, which is an element of *art* and *mathematics*.

Switcheroo!

This body-parts activity is played in pairs, with partners standing back to back. When you call out the name of a body part (or parts), the children turn to face each other, briefly connect those parts, and return to their back-to-back position. When you call out "Switcheroo!" children must get back to back with a new partner; and the game begins again as you call out more body parts.

Possible "connections" to be made include the following:

- hands (both, right, or left)
- knees
- elbows
- feet
- wrists
- right or left shoulders
- right or left hips
- right or left ankles
- big toes
- pointer (ring, baby) fingers

Extending the Activity: This game can be made more challenging by playing it in *trios*. You can also ask children to connect nonmatching body parts (for example, a hand to a knee).

Observation and Evaluation: Does the child properly identify body parts? Does the child work cooperatively with others? Does the child easily identify right from left?

Curriculum Connectors: Body-part identification falls under the heading of *science*, while the cooperative aspect constitutes *social studies*.

Follow the Leader

Follow the Leader is a group activity that provides practice with imitation of movement. If you think your students are ready to handle the responsibility, you should sit this one out and have the children themselves take turns serving as the leader.

Your role in this activity is to stress the best possible imitation and to issue follow-up questions that can help the leader use a variety of movements and spatial patterns. For instance, if the leader is walking only, you can ask if there is another way to move using both feet. How about one foot? Can the leader use his or her arms to make a different body shape? What about a path that does not go around in a circle?

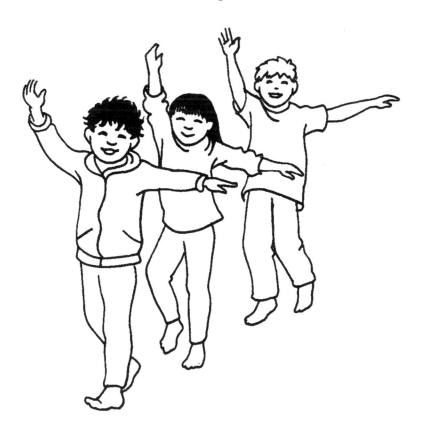

Extending the Activity: In the game Calling Names, performed like Follow the Leader, you will act as leader. The children form a line behind you, and you begin to walk. You then call out the name of one of the children, and she or he breaks away from the line, followed by those behind her or him. This second line begins making its own path around the room.

Continue in this manner, with each new group following its own path while being careful not to intersect another line. It is less confusing if you call the names of children toward the end of the line at first, those who have only a few other children behind them.

Observation and Evaluation: Is the child able to physically replicate movement? Is the child aware and respectful of the personal space of others? Does the child cooperate with a group? Is the child able to lead, demonstrating variety of movement?

Curriculum Connectors: Spatial awareness and physical replication of what the eyes see are components of *art* and *language arts*, while the cooperative nature of the activities fall under the heading of *social studies*.

Pass a Movement

This activity is similar to Pass a Face (see Openers and Closers, page 32) and depends on group cooperation for its success. Standing, form a circle with the children and begin by choosing an action that each child must imitate in his or her turn, until it comes back to you. For instance, you gently squeeze the hand of the child to your right, and he or she must do the same to the child to his or her right, and so on around the circle. Other simple actions follow:

- rising onto tiptoe
- jumping once
- hopping once
- bending at the waist and straightening
- raising and lowering arms

Extending the Activity: Once children grasp the idea, they can take turns starting the action. Every time a movement is returned to the previous leader, the next child in the circle becomes the leader.

To make it more challenging, have each child imitate the movement passed on to her or him, but then also make a *new* movement, which she or he then passes to the next child. In small groups of three to five, each child could be responsible for repeating *all* of the preceding movements before creating one of his or her own.

Observation and Evaluation: Is the child able to imitate the movement being passed? Can the child think of a movement of her or his own? Can the child recall preceding movements?

Curriculum Connectors: Because the movement is passed sequentially around a circle, *mathematics* concepts are addressed. Additionally, the cooperation involved qualifies as *social studies*.

Cooperative Musical Chairs

This game is played much the same as traditional musical chairs, in that the children move around the chairs while music is playing and must get to a chair and sit in it when the music stops. As each round begins, another chair is removed from the game.

The big difference with this game is that children who cannot find a chair to sit in are not eliminated (only to sit and watch the rest of the children continue to have fun). Rather, the goal is for the children to find—and to continue to find—ways they can all fit on the remaining chairs! Even if they all get just one big toe on the last remaining chair, they have all achieved success!

Extending the Activity: More challenging is to limit the ways in which children "fit" onto the remaining chairs with each round. For example, you might ask them to find a way to use only the right side of their bodies for one round, the lower half of the body for another round, and only a "digit" for another.

Observation and Evaluation: Does the child work cooperatively with a group? Is the child successful at problem solving?

Adding Equipment: To make the game less challenging at first, use hoops laid flat on the floor in place of chairs.

Curriculum Connectors: Stopping and starting the music requires children to differentiate between sound and silence, and, of course, because the game is about cooperation, it falls under the heading of *social studies*. To add a *mathematics* element to the game, ask the children to count the original number of chairs and then to tell you the number remaining with each round. Listening is critical to both *music* and *language arts*.

Mirror Game II

In the Mirror Game in Openers and Closers (page 36), you stand before the children and ask them to "reflect" your movements. Here the children are asked to pair off and to stand facing each other. One child performs a series of simple movements (standing in place), which the second child mirrors. After a while, the children reverse roles.

Extending the Activity: Challenge the children to perform a sequence of two or three movements for their partners, which partners must then imitate. Partners can alternate going first.

Observation and Evaluation: Is the child physically able to replicate what the eyes are seeing? Does the child work cooperatively with a partner?

Curriculum Connectors: Being able to physically replicate what the eyes are seeing is a central component of *art*, while the concept of mirror reflections falls under the heading of *science*. The cooperative nature places it under *social studies*.

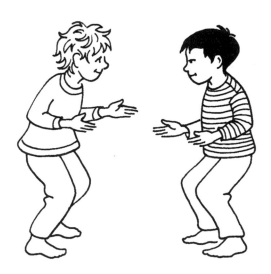

Shadow Game

As this activity is based on the concept of shadows, you might want to talk to the children about shadows before beginning this activity. This is a partner activity, similar to the Mirror Game and played in pairs. With this game, one child stands with her or his back to the second child and performs various movements that the partner standing behind "shadows." Then they trade roles. These should all be performed with the children standing in one place.

Extending the Activity: When the children are ready, invite them to perform the activity while moving around the room as person and shadow. Again, they should switch roles. Encourage variety in their movement by suggesting different body shapes, pathways, levels, directions, and tempos.

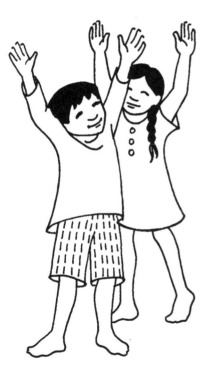

Observation and Evaluation: Is the child able to physically replicate what the eyes are seeing? Does the child work cooperatively with a partner?

Curriculum Connectors: The cooperative nature of these activities place them under *social studies*, while the concept of shadows belongs to *science*. Being able to physically replicate what the eyes see is essential to both *art* and *language arts* (writing).

Circle Design

Ask the children to form a circle and lightly join hands. They then place one foot inside the circle and one to the back in order to plant themselves firmly in place. Without moving their feet or losing hand contact (they are allowed to turn their hands within one another's), they should experiment with changing the design of the circle. For example, the circle might go from the middle level (standing) to a low level (anything lower than standing), or every other child could move to a low level. The group can also experiment with changing the round shape of the circle. (*Note:* Stress the fact that the point of the activity is to see how many designs are possible given the restrictions imposed—not to throw one another off balance! If your class is very large, you may want to separate the children into smaller groups.)

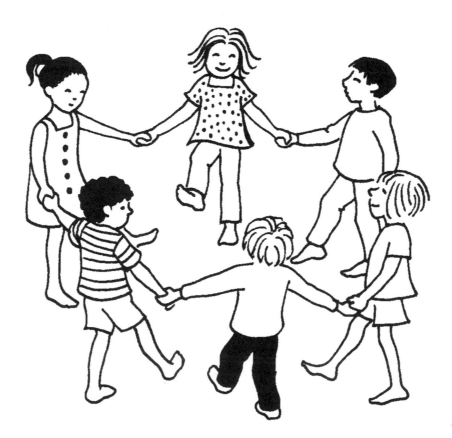

Extending the Activity: Once your students have experimented successfully with this, challenge each of them to free one foot and see how that changes the possible designs. Finally, you can ask them to free both feet, with hands still joined.

Observation and Evaluation: Does the child cooperate effectively with the group? Does the child contribute ideas? Does the child understand the concept involved?

Curriculum Connectors: In addition to an experience in *social studies*, these activities offer additional practice with the concept of shape, which is central to *art* and geometry (*mathematics*).

Palm to Palm

In this partner activity, the children pair off and face each other, standing about a foot apart. The first child then places his or her arms into any position, with palms flat and facing the partner. The partner quickly places his or her palms against the first child's so they lightly touch. Once contact is made, the first child quickly assumes a new arm position, and the activity continues in this manner. After a while partners reverse roles.

Extending the Activity: Initially, children are likely to assume symmetrical arm positions (both arms identical). Once they have had some experience with this, encourage them to find asymmetrical solutions as well (for example, one arm high and the other low).

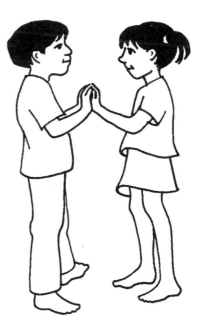

Observation and Evaluation: Can the child isolate one arm from the other? Does the child work cooperatively with a partner? How creative is the child in finding arm positions?

Curriculum Connectors: Because this game is an exploration of shape and is a cooperative activity, it falls under the headings of *art* and *social studies*.

Forming Shapes with Partners

Ask the children to pair off, and then assign shapes that can easily be made by two people. Possible shapes include the following:

a square   a table

a triangle   a chair

a rectangle   a rug

a circle

Extending the Activity: Is forming the above shapes with a *trio* easier or harder? Also, you can assign partners to try more challenging forms. Possibilities include:

pointed   perpendicular

angular   parallel

crooked

Observation and Evaluation: Does the child cooperate effectively with a partner? Is the child familiar with the shape? Can the child replicate the shape with a partner?

Curriculum Connectors: Shape in general falls under the heading of *art*, while the geometric shapes specifically are linked to *mathematics*. Also, the cooperative nature of the activities places them under *social studies*.

Forming Letters with Partners

Begin the activity by discussing the difference between the straight, curving, and angular lines that make up letters. You may wish to have the children demonstrate with their bodies the three different types of lines. Ask the children to pair off, and then assign letters that they can easily form with two people. Possibilities include A, H, O, D, P, J, L, S, T, V, W, and Y.

Extending the Activity: Similarly, you can ask children to pair off and form numbers. Possibilities include 2, 3, 4, 6, 7, 8, 9, and 10.

Observation and Evaluation: Does the child realistically replicate *letters* and *numbers*? Does the child differentiate among straight, curving, and angular lines?

Adding Equipment: Provide large letters on poster board for children to follow. An alternative activity is to invite partners to create various letters and numbers with a rope on the floor, and then to replicate the shape with their bodies. They can also follow the pathways created by the shape with a variety of locomotor skills.

Curriculum Connectors: The concept of line is central to *art* and early geometry (*mathematics*). Letters, of course, fall under *language arts* and numbers under *mathematics*, while the cooperative nature of the activities places them under *social studies*.

Touch and Move

This is a partner activity that requires a lot of respect and cooperation between partners, but the children should be ready to give it a try.

The activity asks pairs of students to connect various body parts, which you designate, and then discover how many ways they can move, despite the limitation. Instruct the children to pair off and then to connect the following parts:

right or left hands	backs
right or left elbows	right or left shoulders
one or both knees	noses
right or left feet	both hands and both
tops of heads	feet

Extending the Activity: Challenge children to connect *nonmatching* parts, like a hand and an elbow, a hand and a knee, or a shoulder and a back!

Observation and Evaluation: Is the child able to stay "connected"? Does the child discover a variety of ways to move?

Curriculum Connectors: This game requires a great deal of problem solving, which is critical to learning in all areas, including *social studies*, addressed by the cooperative nature of the game. The concept of "how many" is quantitative and therefore *mathematics*.

Matching Shapes

Separate the class into two equal-sized groups, assigning one group to be *ones* and the other *twos*. Then instruct the *ones* to begin walking around the room on your signal to go. When you call out a shape (for example, crooked, narrow, wide, round, flat, small, tall, pointed, and so on), each child must stop, assume a version of that shape, and hold the pose. Each *two* must then choose a child from the *ones* (you may decide to prearrange partners), stand before that child, and assume the same shape. The *ones* then look on as you give the signal for the *twos* to begin walking around the room, and the process continues.

Extending the Activity: To play Shapes in Motion, ask the children to pair off. The first child forms a shape and, remaining in that shape, moves toward the second child. For example, if the child is in a small rounded shape on the floor, he or she could roll toward the second child. The second child then goes over, under, or around the first, depending on the possibilities involved. (In the example given, the second child might leap over the first as he or she is rolling.) The second child then becomes the first child, assuming a new shape of his or her own.

Observation and Evaluation: Is the child able to create his or her own version of the shape you call out, without imitating others? Is the child able to match a partner's shape? Does the child find ways to move while in a particular shape? Can the child discover ways to move over, under, or around a partner?

Curriculum Connectors: Because cooperative activities teach lessons about being and working together, they can be considered *social studies*. Shape is a central component of *art* and *mathematics*. Matching is also a mathematics concept, and the ability to physically replicate what the eyes see is part of both art and *language arts*.

Moving Forward with a Partner

The children have had quite a bit of partner work at this point, so they understand the cooperation required, and that's good, because they are about to discover that even simple locomotor skills can have different requirements when performed with a partner.

Ask the children to pair off, and explain that they are going to execute a variety of movements in a forward direction, linked to their partners in a variety of ways. Locomotor skills you can suggest include the following:

- walk
- run
- gallop
- skip
- jump

Partners can try the previous locomotor skills with the following:

- inside hands joined
- inside arms linked
- right and left hands joined, with arms crossed
- arms around each other's waists
- inside hands on each other's shoulders
- right hands joined with one partner's arm across the other partner's shoulders and left hands joined in front

Extending the Activity: Repeat the above activity, with the exception of the gallop, challenging partners to link in a variety of ways moving *backward*. Remind them to look behind themselves first and then to proceed with caution.

The next step is to challenge partners to move while *facing each other*. Possible contacts include the following:

- hands held in front
- hands held and extended to sides

- arms crossed in front and opposite hands held
- the waist-shoulder social dance position, with one partner's hands on the other's waist and the second partner's hands on the other's shoulders

Observation and Evaluation: Is the child able to perform the locomotor skill with a partner as well as he or she can individually? Can the child coordinate and synchronize her or his movements to those of a partner? Is the child successful with each of the contacts?

Curriculum Connectors: Because rhythm and synchronized movement are essential to these exercises, they fall under the heading of *music* and *language arts*. The cooperative nature of the activities makes them part of *social studies*.

Ducks, Cows, Cats, and Dogs

In this activity, the children play different animals. The object is for like animals to find one another. Ask the children to space themselves evenly throughout the room. Then whisper the name of one of the animals in the title in each player's ear (the easiest way is to simply say them in the same order over and over again). Once all the children have been assigned an animal, they close their eyes and get on hands and knees. Tell them that without talking, they are to find all the other animals like themselves. At your start signal, the "animals" begin to move, making the appropriate sounds.

When they have found other animals like themselves, they stop making their sounds and sit and watch the others who are still trying. Help the children by letting them know when all of the cats, for example, have found each other.

Extending the Activity: To make the game more challenging, add other animals with familiar sounds, like pigs, chickens, or sheep.

Observation and Evaluation: Does the child keep his or her eyes closed? Does the child exhibit the listening skills necessary for finding his or her matching animal? Is the child able to avoid collisions with others?

Adding Equipment: If the children are feeling particularly brave, you can avoid the temptation to "peek" by placing a blindfold on each child.

Curriculum Connectors: Because this is a listening—or sound discrimination—activity, it falls under the headings of *music* and *language arts*. Focus on animals adds a *science* element, while the cooperation qualifies as *social studies*. Once all the "animals" have found each other, ask the children to count the numbers in each group, contributing a *mathematics* experience. To incorporate *art* (and therefore touch on all content areas!), invite the children to draw their assigned animals.

Synchronized Partners

Have the children work in pairs. One partner begins by choosing a movement that he or she repeats continuously. In the meantime, the second partner chooses a different movement that interrelates but does not interfere with the movement of the first child.

For example, the first child may choose to rock back and forth. The second child walks around the first, timing her or his walk to avoid the rocking of the first child. Another example would be if the first child were to wave her or his arms up and down. The second child might choose to move around the first, timing the movement so as to pass under the first child's arms as they are raised. (*Note:* If the children have difficulty deciding on their own movements at first, you can offer suggestions similar to those described in the previous paragraph.)

Extending the Activity: Once children have the knack of synchronization in partners, it is time for them to build a machine! One child begins by repeatedly performing a movement that can be executed in one spot. A second child then stands near the first and contributes a second movement that relates in some way to the first. For example, if the first child is performing an up-down motion by bending and stretching, the second child might choose to do the reverse, standing beside her or his classmate. A third child is then added, performing a movement of his or her own.

The movements of the first three children continue as each remaining child adds a new functioning "part" to the machine. Once all the parts are functioning, ask the children to each make a sound that corresponds to her or his movement.

Observation and Evaluation: Does the child understand the concept of synchronization? Does the child cooperate effectively with a partner and with a group? Is the child able to discover responses of his or her own?

Curriculum Connectors: The cooperative nature of these activities falls under the heading of *social studies*, while the concepts of synchronization and machinery can be considered *science* concepts.

Turning with a Partner

Once the children have achieved success moving forward and backward with a partner (page 117), they can experiment with turning as they perform the walk, run, and skip.

As before, partners should link up in the following ways as they explore possibilities. Also, they should be facing in different directions in order to turn around. Possible connections are as follows:

- inside hands joined
- inside arms linked
- right and left hands joined, with arms crossed
- arms around each other's waists
- inside hands on each other's shoulders
- right hands joined in back, with one partner's arm across the other partner's shoulders, and left hands joined in front

Extending the Activity: What possibilities can partners discover while *facing* each other? Students can chart possibilities and record whether or not they work.

Observation and Evaluation: Does the child cooperate effectively with a partner? Is the child able to turn with a partner in each of the positions, using each of the physical connections? Does the child discover new possibilities?

Curriculum Connectors: The cooperation involved places these activities under the heading of *social studies*. The experimentation involved contributes an aspect of *science*, with charting and recording possibilities bringing in *mathematics*.

Footsie Rolls

Discuss log rolls with the children (see Let's Roll II, page 137). Then have them pair off, with partners lying on their backs with the soles of their feet together. The object in this activity is for the partners to roll over without their feet breaking contact. This one takes lots of cooperation and enough room to move safely. For example, if you have a small area for movement, you may be limited to only one or two sets of partners working at a time. Any waiting children can act as the audience, cheering or applauding while the partners remain connected and groaning when the connection is broken. Once the connection is broken, another pair takes a turn.

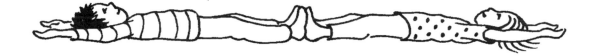

Extending the Activity: Increasing the challenge can include asking partners to roll from one end of the room to the other, and in both directions.

Observation and Evaluation: Does the child work cooperatively with a partner? Is the child able to roll with a straight body, in a straight pathway? Is the child able to coordinate her or his movements with those of a partner?

Curriculum Connectors: Rolling requires impetus and momentum, which are *science* concepts. Cooperative activities, of course, qualify as *social studies*.

Let's Slither

This is an exercise requiring a lot of cooperation among the children.

The students begin by pairing off and stretching out on their stomachs, one in front of the other. The child in back takes hold of the ankles of the child in front, forming a two-person "snake" that starts to slither across the floor. After a while, partners reverse leads.

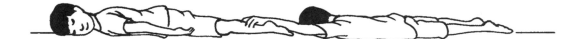

Extending the Activity: Once children demonstrate they are able to slither smoothly in pairs, challenge each two-person snake to connect with another two-person snake, with the process continuing until the entire group has formed one big snake!

Observation and Evaluation: Does the child cooperate effectively with a partner and in a group? Is the child able to follow (lead) in this activity? Is the child able to slither?

Curriculum Connectors: A discussion about snakes and other creatures that slither can contribute some *science* to these activities. Cooperation falls under the heading of *social studies*.

Exploring Contrasts

Previously, the children explored opposites (see Exploring Opposites, page 75). In this activity, they will explore the concept of contrasts.

Have the children pair off. Ask the first of each pair to move in one of the following ways, and the second to move in a contrasting way. Initially, you should assign the contrast. The children take turns being first.

Possible contrasts include the following:

- a whisper (movement); a shout (contrast)
- a gentle breeze (movement); a gale wind (contrast)
- a torrent of rain (movement); a sprinkle (contrast)
- a pebble rolling down a hill (movement); a boulder crashing down a mountain (contrast)
- a raging fire (movement); a flickering candle (contrast)

Extending the Activity: Once children grasp the idea involved, allow them to decide for themselves what the contrast should be. You can also include more abstract concepts, such as the following possibilities:

- classical music (movement); hard rock (contrast)
- a horror movie (movement); a comedy (contrast)

Observation and Evaluation: Does the child understand the concept of contrasts? Is the child able to depict the contrast through movement?

Curriculum Connectors: The cooperation involved makes this a lesson in *social studies*. The concept of contrasts contributes a *language arts* experience. The contrasts also explore the movement element of force (light versus strong), which are quantitative concepts under the heading of *mathematics*.

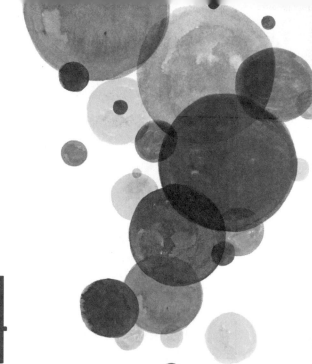

UNIT 4

Educational Gymnastics

Included in this section are activities related to the gymnastic skills of transferring weight, rolling, and balancing. Also included in this unit is the exploration of combinations of locomotor and nonlocomotor skills, as gymnastics typically involves the sequencing of movement skills.

Locomotion

Challenge the children to imitate an animal that walks on four legs. Can it also walk backward? Ask them to show you a smaller animal, and then a larger one, both of which also walk on four legs. How does a seal move? (Desired goal: lying prone, legs straight behind, arms held straight and used to move body forward; legs dragging.) An inchworm? (Goal: lying in a push-up position, taking a few small "steps" forward with hands. Leaving hands where they are, feet are moved forward until they reach hands.)

Extending the Activity: Invite the children to try walking with hands placed on their knees. Once they have accomplished this, challenge them to try walking with their hands on their ankles. Can they do it backward and sideways as well? How many other ways can they find to walk? Are there ways that do not involve the feet?

Observation and Evaluation: Is the child able to respond to the challenges without the teacher demonstrating the movement(s)? Does the child show the upper body strength required to move like a seal or an inchworm? Which of the challenges require repetition?

Curriculum Connectors: Exploration of the way in which various creatures move constitutes *science*.

Moving with Limitations

This exercise requires the children to give some thought to the way in which they move because it places restrictions on their responses.

Pose the following challenges, giving the children ample opportunity to experiment with one before moving on to another:

- Show me you can move while being very small. Very round. Very narrow.
- Think of a way to move using both your hands and feet.
- Show me you can move without using your feet at all.
- Think of a way to move your body very close to the floor. Find another way.
- Not including your feet, how many parts of your body can you walk on? Can you walk while kneeling? While sitting?
- Move by using your feet but not for walking. Find another way.

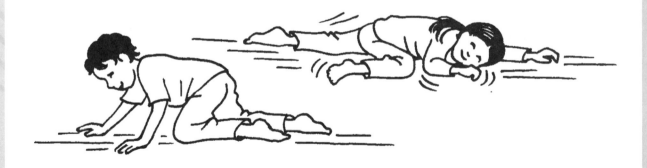

Extending the Activity: You can make the activity even more challenging by asking your students to find *how many* ways they can move given a particular limitation. Because this is a broader request than those made previously, you will want to give the children more time to discover a variety of responses.

Pose the following questions and challenges:

- Place your hands on the floor and show me how many ways you can move your feet (without moving your hands).
- Can you find different ways to move if you have just one hand on the floor?
- Try it with one foot and both hands. How many ways can you move the free foot?
- Put the top of your head on the floor and find how many ways you can move the rest of your body.

Observation and Evaluation: Does the child respond to the initial challenges? Is the child able to find more than one way to respond to the later challenges?

Curriculum Connectors: "How many" is a quantitative concept falling under the heading of *mathematics*. Experimentation, of course, is central to *science*, as is the identification of body parts and their use.

Jumping and Landing

Challenge the children to perform the following tasks:

- Blast off: Squat low, pretending to be a spaceship on the launching pad. At the end of the countdown, blast off.
- Frog jump: A frog uses front and back legs at the same time to push off the ground but lands with the hind feet first.
- Knee slap: At the height of the jump, knees are drawn toward the chest and slapped. Then can they slap one knee at a time? Cross arms and slap opposite knees?

Extending the Activity: More challenging are the following:

- Seat kicker: Jump upward, bending knees and kicking backward, "get the feet to meet the seat."
- Star jump: Jump with a star body shape, with arms and legs spread out, and land in a balanced, stable position.
- Tuck jump: At the height of the jump, knees are drawn toward the chest. Grasp shins, back straight.

Observation and Evaluation: In all cases, does the child land with knees bent and heels coming all the way to the floor? Which of the challenges is the child able to meet, and which require additional practice?

Curriculum Connectors: A discussion about why we are not able to stay in the air when we jump (because of gravity) can incorporate a *science* element.

Exploring Weight Placement

In this exercise, the children are going to experiment with the placement of weight on various body parts. You can explain the placement of weight by telling them that only the body parts you assign will be touching the floor.

Ask them to place only the following body parts on the floor:

hands and knees	one side of the body;
knees and elbows	the other
knees alone	just the bottom
just the tummy	hands and feet
the back	just the feet

Extending the Activity: Once children are familiar with this concept, add weight transferal to the activity, explaining that you want them first to put only those body parts you assign on the floor and then to shift the next body parts assigned as *smoothly* as possible.

Observation and Evaluation: Is the child able to place his or her weight on only those body parts assigned? Can the child transfer weight smoothly from one position to the next?

Curriculum Connectors: Experimentation with weight placement and transferal qualifies as *science* for young children.

Counting Body Parts

This exercise is similar to the previous activity, Exploring Weight Placement, in which you assigned body parts for the placement of weight. This time, however, you will simply give the children a *number* of body parts on which to place their weight, letting them choose the parts themselves.

Ask the children to place their weight on five, four, three, two, and one body part(s) at a time, challenging them to find at least two solutions to each combination (for example, a challenge to place weight on one part only could result in standing on the right or left foot, sitting on the bottom, or balancing on one or the other knee).

Extending the Activity: During repetitions of this activity, challenge the children to find *as many solutions as possible* to each combination. If necessary, remind them to try these challenges at low, middle, and high levels.

Observation and Evaluation: This is a simple way to assess whether or not the child is having difficulty with counting. Also, is the child able to find more than one solution to each challenge?

Curriculum Connectors: Counting, of course, is a component of *mathematics*. Because balance and stability are also involved in these exercises, they offer experiences in *science* too.

Static Balance

· ·

Balance is a necessary skill for everyone. In these activities, the children will become familiar with the concept of static balance at both low and high levels in space. Unlike the previous two activities in this unit, the goal here is not simply to place weight on the assigned body parts but actually to *balance* on them and only them. As you issue the following challenges, remind your students that they are just going to see how these balances feel, as you cannot expect them to master all of the balances yet.

Ask them to try the following low-level balances:

on two hands and one
   knee
on one hand and one
   knee

on bottom only
on knees only
on tummy only
on one knee

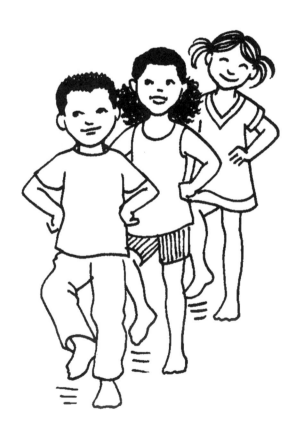

Extending the Activity: The next step is to suggest high-level balances like the following:

on tiptoe	on tiptoe with eyes
on one foot (flat)	closed
on the other foot	on one foot, on tiptoe
on tiptoe with knees bent	

All of the challenges below are preceded with a rise onto tiptoe. Ask the children to get on tiptoe; then pose the following challenges and questions:

- How long can you stay up there?
- Lower your heels in four slow counts. (Slowly count 1-2-3-4.)
- Turn your head to the right; left.
- Close your eyes.
- Slowly lift one foot off the floor and bring it to the side of your knee on the supporting leg. Try it with your other leg.

Observation and Evaluation: Is the child able to balance at a low level, on all assigned body parts? Can the child balance at a high level? Does the child have greater success with some of the latter challenges than others?

Adding Equipment: For the initial high-level challenges, children may experience greater success if they are holding onto something, such as a parachute.

Curriculum Connectors: Balance is a *science* concept, while low and high are relevant to both *art* and *mathematics*.

Sitting Balances

Challenge your students to try the following "balances on the bottom":

- Tuck sit: Sit with knees bent and near chest. Balance on buttocks with toes resting on the floor. Hold for three seconds.
- Straddle sit: Sit with legs straddled and upper body stretched upward at 90 degrees to the legs. Arms are straight and stretched overhead, shoulder-width apart. Raise legs off floor and balance on the buttocks for three seconds.
- Sit and spin: Sit with legs bent, hands on floor. Lift the feet off the floor and use your hands to spin the body. Tightly tuck and wrap hands around knees. Stay seated (don't fall back)!

Extending the Activity: More challenging is the V-sit, which begins as a tuck sit. One at a time, the legs are then raised off the floor and extended, in the shape of a V, in front of the body. Can the children achieve this from a straddle sit? Can they sit and spin in this position?

Observation and Evaluation: Does the child possess the balance and abdominal strength required of these balances? Is the child able to sit and spin without falling over?

Curriculum Connectors: Balance is a *science* concept.

Dynamic Balance

· ·

Ask students to find—or imagine—a straight line on the floor. Then, pretending they are tightrope walkers, they should move across the line in the following ways:

- forward
- sideways
- backward
- forward on tiptoe
- backward on tiptoe

Extending the Activity: Next, challenge them to perform the following locomotor skills across their "tightropes":

run	hop
gallop	leap
slide	skip

Which of these can be executed backward and/or sideways?

Finally, ask them to create a routine they might perform in the circus. The routine should take them from one end of the tightrope to the other and include at least two forms of locomotion and two different directions.

Observation and Evaluation: Does the child understand the concept of placing one foot before the other to stay "on the tightrope"? Is the child able to move in all directions, executing all of the locomotor skills?

Adding Equipment: Placing a jump rope or masking tape on the floor can help make these challenges less abstract. Also, all of the above challenges can later be executed on a low balance beam. With the latter, you can issue additional challenges for the children to discover how many ways they can find to travel both over and along the beam.

Curriculum Connectors: Balance is a *science* concept. Any discussion of the lives and work of real-life tightrope walkers can make *social studies* part of the activity.

Let's Roll I

Challenge the children to perform the following rolls:

- Egg roll: Sit with feet flat on floor, knees bent toward chest and apart, hands grasping the ankles. Roll from one side to the other, across the shoulders, and back to a sitting position.
- Puppy dog roll: Kneel with hands on the ground. Sit back onto legs. Roll 180 degrees, contacting the ground at shoulder, hip, and back. Stay in a tucked position throughout.
- Roll-arounds: Sit in a straddle position, legs wide apart and slightly bent. Grasp the legs as close to the ankles as possible. Roll to one shoulder, across the back to the other, and back up to a sitting position. (*Hint:* Roll-arounds are most successfully performed when momentum is built, allowing for smooth, continuous motion.)

Extending the Activity: More challenging is a series involving the back rocker. Invite your students to try the following:

- Back rocker: Sit in a tucked position with back rounded and chin near chest. Rock backward and forward. Execute a back rocker and then use hands to push off floor to feet, finishing in a T-stand, with arms extended to sides.
- From stand to back rocker: Start standing tall with arms forward horizontally. Sit, using hands for support. Rock back and forth without stopping.
- Back rocker with hand touch: Sit in a tucked position, back rounded and chin on chest. Place hands by ears, palms upward and backward. Rock backward and forward, hands touching the floor behind the head each time.

Observation and Evaluation: Does the child execute each roll correctly? Which require additional practice?

Curriculum Connectors: Each of these rolls requires a different body shape, and shape is a component of *art* and *mathematics*. The momentum and motion of a roll fall under the heading of *science*.

Let's Roll II

A roll is generally defined as a movement made by a body that is *supine* (face up) or *prone* (face down) and fully extended, with the arms stretched overhead. Ask the children to experiment with this type of roll, often called a "log roll," making sure they roll in both directions, both slowly and quickly.

Extending the Activity: Once the children are experiencing success with log rolls, challenge them to initiate a roll with first the upper torso and then the lower torso. (The body will start out "crooked" but then straighten.)

Observation and Evaluation: Is the child able to roll with a straight body, in a straight pathway? Can the child perform the roll in both directions? Can the child initiate the roll with the upper and lower torsos?

Adding Equipment: To help the children actually see whether or not they are rolling in straight pathways, you can create a wide "lane" by setting up two rows of plastic cones.

Curriculum Connectors: Rolling is a simple *science* concept.

Symmetrical and Asymmetrical Balances

Ask students to begin in a V-sit (balancing on bottom with arms out to sides and legs lifted and extended in a straddle to front). Explain that since both sides of the body look exactly the same, this is a symmetrical balance. Now issue the following challenges:

- While still maintaining balance on your seat, change the position of your arms to create another symmetrical shape.
- Create another symmetrical shape by changing the position of your legs.
- Create an asymmetrical shape. Another.
- Create a symmetrical shape with arms and legs, but then change the position of your head so the overall shape is asymmetrical.
- Practice moving smoothly from a symmetrical balance to an asymmetrical one and back again.

Extending the Activity: Challenge partners to create a short sequence that moves from a symmetrical balance to an asymmetrical one and back again. In both of these balances, they must use one another for support, and both partners must alter their positions to change from one balance to the other.

Observation and Evaluation: Does the child understand the concepts of symmetrical and asymmetrical? Is the child able to demonstrate both kinds of balances? Does the child cooperate effectively with a partner in the extended activity?

Curriculum Connectors: Balance is a *science* concept, while symmetrical and asymmetrical shapes fall under the heading of *art* and *mathematics*. The cooperative nature of the extension activity places it under *social studies*.

Balance and Recovery

Challenge the students to achieve balances, using the bases of support listed below. In each of these balances, they are to see how far they can lean before falling over. They then return to their original positions. Encourage them to lean forward, backward, right, and left.

Possible bases of support include:

both feet (flat)   one foot on tiptoe

both feet on tiptoe   both knees

one foot (flat)   one knee

on tiptoe with knees bent   the bottom

on tiptoe with eyes closed

Extending the Activity: Designate a certain number of counts (beginning with eight) during which students must lean and then recover (as you are counting aloud, they use all eight counts to lean as far as they can; you then begin counting again, and they use the next eight counts to move back into their original positions). This can be made even more challenging by decreasing the number of counts until the students are asked to balance and recover in just two counts each!

Observation and Evaluation: Does the child understand the concept of balance and recovery? Is the child able to stop before leaning too far? Does the child have the balance necessary to recover original positions?

Curriculum Connectors: Balance is a *science* concept. Counting and time are components of *mathematics*.

Partner Balance

Ask the children to work with a partner, and then challenge each pair to achieve and maintain a balance that could not be achieved by just one person. For example, one partner provides support while the other stands on one foot and leans against her or him. How many possibilities can they find?

Extending the Activity: Challenge the children to find a balance in which one partner acts as a base and the second balances on that base, getting his or her weight completely off the floor. Watch this one for safety!

Observation and Evaluation: Does the child cooperate effectively with a partner? Does the child contribute ideas to the process? Does the child maintain successful balances?

Adding Equipment: Give each pair of students a hoop and challenge them to find how many ways they can achieve balances incorporating the prop.

Curriculum Connectors: Balance is a *science* concept, while the cooperative nature of these activities constitutes *social studies*.

More Partner Balances

This activity explores the concept of counterbalance.

Challenge partners to discover how many ways they can *push* against each other to achieve a balance, encouraging them to explore different levels and to push with a variety of body parts. Do they always have to use matching body parts to achieve a balance?

Now ask partners to explore *pulling away* from each other in order to achieve a balance. Again, encourage them also to try *nonmatching* body parts.

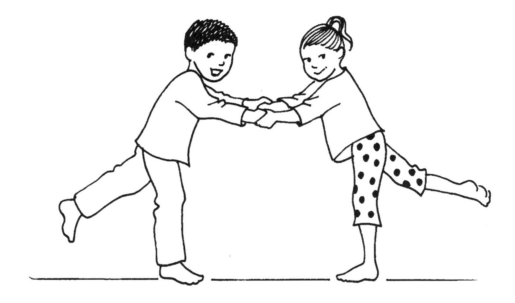

Extending the Activity: When students are ready, ask them to achieve a balance, with their stability dependent upon one another, and to experiment with how many ways they can move while still maintaining their balance. For example, if partners were both standing on one foot on tiptoe, clasping each other's hands above their heads, they might raise and lower their bodies or hop in different directions. Because they are moving, their solutions will be dynamic counterbalances.

Observation and Evaluation: Does the child cooperate effectively with a partner? Does the child understand the concept of counterbalance? Is the child able to achieve counterbalances?

Curriculum Connectors: Balance is a *science* concept, and cooperation falls under *social studies.*

Group Balance

Ask the children to form a circle and to place their hands on the shoulders of the children beside them. Explain that the object of this exercise is to maintain a steady balance. Then issue the following challenges:

- Rise onto tiptoe.
- Rise onto tiptoe and bend your knees.
- Stand on the right foot only (flat). Try rising onto tiptoe.
- Stand on the left foot only. Rise onto tiptoe on that foot.
- Stand on just one foot and extend the free leg into the center of the circle.
- Rise onto tiptoe and bend forward at the waist.

Extending the Activity: Put the students' problem-solving skills to work by challenging them to discover how many other ways they can find to balance as a group. (*Hint:* They do not have to remain in a circle.)

Observation and Evaluation: Does the child attempt to meet the objective of contributing to a group balance? Is the child able to maintain balance in all positions? Does the child contribute ideas to the extension activity?

Adding Equipment: As an alternative to standing with hands on shoulders, students can attempt a group balance while gathered around a parachute.

Curriculum Connectors: In addition to the *social studies* aspect of this cooperative activity, the children are gaining experience with balance, which is a *science* concept. "How many" is a quantitative concept under the content area of *mathematics*.

Exploring Upside Down

Many gymnastics activities involve upside-down positions. However, because your children are likely to be at varying levels of gymnastic ability, this activity is intended to give every student a chance to participate at his or her own level. Stress the fact that the children are to simply *experiment* with upside-down activities so they do not feel pressured into trying things they may not yet be ready for. (*Note:* These exercises require a carpeted or matted surface.)

This exploration uses a process of convergent problem solving that guides students to their discoveries. Pose the following questions and challenges to the children:

- Show me an upside-down position.
- Show me you can be upside down with your weight on four body parts. Find another way.
- Show me an upside-down position with your weight on five body parts.
- In that position, see if you can raise one hand off the floor. Is it possible to raise both hands off? One hand and one foot? Can you lift a hand on one side and a foot on the opposite side?

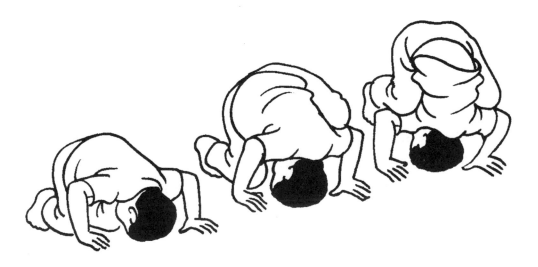

Extending the Activity: Following are more difficult challenges that should eventually lead to execution of a tripod formation:

- With your weight on five body parts, put one knee on top of the elbow on that side. Try it on the other side. Let your knees take turns climbing up on your elbows. (*Note:* The elbows will provide more stability if they are pressed inward rather than outward.)
- Try putting both knees up on your elbows so your weight is on just three body parts. (When accomplished, the result is a tripod, the first step in performing a headstand.) How long can you stay that way?

Should children master the tripod, you can further challenge them to extend one leg at a time, first behind them and then straight above.

Observation and Evaluation: How many of these challenges is the child able to manage? Does the child show apprehension concerning upside-down positions? Does the child understand the challenges?

Curriculum Connectors: Spatial awareness falls under the heading of *art* but is also essential to *language arts*. Counting body parts is a *mathematics* experience, and balance a *science* experience.

Discovering the Forward Roll

This activity again uses a process of convergent problem solving, this time leading the children toward the discovery of a forward roll. Present the following challenges:

- Show me an upside-down position. (If necessary, follow up with: Show me an upside-down position with weight on the hands and feet. And, if necessary: Show me an upside-down position with weight on the hands and feet and the tummy facing the floor.)
- Look behind yourself from that upside-down position. Look at the ceiling. Show me you can look at even more of the ceiling.
- With your chin tucked to your chest, roll yourself over from that position. (A forward roll is the hoped-for result.) Can you do it more than once?

Extending the Activity: Once the children have mastered the forward roll, the next challenge is to finish the roll in a sitting position, legs straight on the floor. More challenging still is to finish standing, arms extended to sides (called a T-stand).

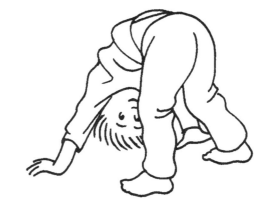

Observation and Evaluation: Is the child discovering a forward roll? Can the child properly, and thus, safely, execute a forward roll? Is the child able to finish a forward roll, first in a sit and then in a T-stand?

Curriculum Connectors: The gravity and momentum involved in rolling places these activities under *science*. Spatial awareness is central to *art* and *language arts*.

Combining Locomotor Skills

On their way to learning how to master gymnastic skills and sequences, children need to learn how to link together the individual skills they have acquired to form movement "phrases," "sentences," and eventually "paragraphs."

In this exercise, you will suggest combinations of locomotor skills to the children, and they will put them together to form movement phrases. The only stipulation is that the skills be linked without lengthy pauses or any extraneous movements between them. The children may perform as many repeats as they want of each individual skill.

Suggest the following combinations to the children, and give them plenty of time to explore possibilities:

walk-hop-slide   walk-leap-hop

gallop-jump-hop   gallop-leap-run

skip-hop-walk   run-jump-leap

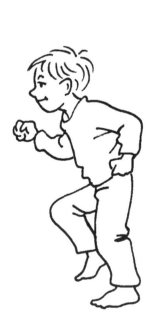
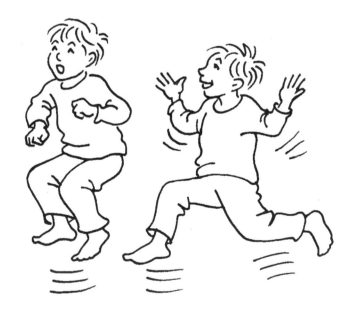

Extending the Activity: Ask the children to explore the possibilities involved in combining locomotor and nonlocomotor skills. Present the following combinations to the students, giving them enough time to explore one before moving on to the next.

Suggested combinations are as follows:

- walk-turn-jump
- stretch-hop-run
- stretch-swing-jump
- skip-sway-slide
- hop-sit-roll
- leap-twist-skip

Observation and Evaluation: Is the child able to perform the individual movement skills? Can the child link them together smoothly?

Curriculum Connectors: The concept of phrases falls under the heading of *language arts*.

Movement Words

Like the preceding activity, this exercise allows children to link movements together to create "phrases." This time, however, the movements are subject to greater interpretation. And the children may link them in any order they choose, once again repeating them as many times as they like and linking them without extraneous movements in between.

Tell the children what the words are and establish a signal that indicates when it is time to change from one to the other. At the sight, or sound, of the signal, the children perform the action in any manner they choose. Repeat this several times, but not so many times that the children become bored.

Begin with simple combinations such as *walking and stretching* and *hopping and bending*. Then challenge students to link all four together.

Extending the Activity: Invite students to try these combinations without the signal from you, allowing them to change from one to the other whenever they choose. Other possible combinations, subject to greater interpretation, include the following:

- rising, falling, and expanding
- shrinking, expanding, and rising
- falling, curling, and stretching

Observation and Evaluation: Does the child link the movements smoothly? Is the child able to interpret the words without imitating anyone else?

Curriculum Connectors: The creation of "phrases" is relative to *language arts*, as is the word comprehension involved.

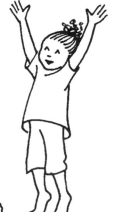

Gymnastic Sequences

This lesson plan requires that the children link movements together, as in the two preceding activities. This time, however, the movements are very gymnastics oriented. The students should start by combining the movements in the order given, again performing them without extraneous transitional movements. Note that these sequences, unlike those in the previous two lesson plans, do not include repetitions of each movement.

Giving students plenty of time to practice each sequence, present the following sequences:

- jump-fall-roll
- run-jump-fall-roll
- balance-fall-roll
- fall-roll-balance
- roll-balance-stretch-curl-pose

Extending the Activity: Challenge students to create their own gymnastic sequences, including opening and closing poses, practicing them until they can perform them exactly the same way each time.

Observation and Evaluation: Is the child able to perform each of the individual movements? Can the child link the movements smoothly?

Adding Equipment: Challenge students to perform their gymnastic sequences on a jump rope stretched out on the floor or on a low balance beam. An additional challenge is to perform these sequences while holding a ribbon stick or ball, as seen in rhythmic gymnastics.

Curriculum Connectors: Balancing and rolling are *science* concepts, while the creation of "phrases" and "sentences" falls under the heading of *language arts*.

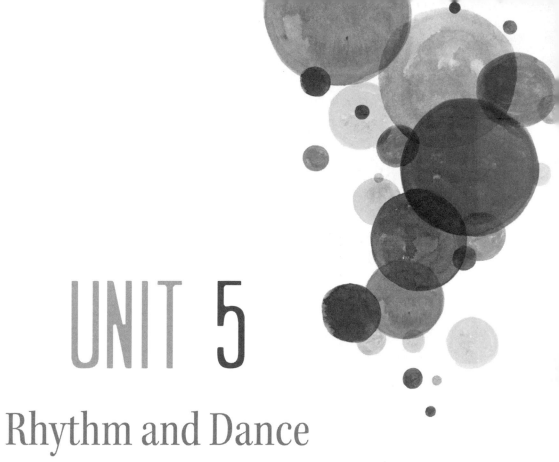

UNIT 5

Rhythm and Dance

The movement element of rhythm, the musical concepts of beat and meter, and the qualities of swinging, sustained, suspended, percussive, vibratory, and collapsing movement are explored in this unit. The Statues game (page 158) offers students the opportunity to improvise and express themselves to a variety of music, and the More Movement Words (page 168) activities provide a chance for students to perform combinations of skills in interpretive and expressive ways. All of the activities in this unit prepare children for dance experiences in the upper elementary grades.

Body Sounds

Ask the children to show you how many different sounds they can create with their bodies. Body parts capable of making sounds include hands, feet, mouth, tongue, and teeth. How do these sounds make them feel like moving?

Extending the Activity: Ask the children to show you how the following words and sounds make them feel like moving:

- Boom! Boom! Boom!
- tweet-tweet
- dum-de-dum-dum
- la-di-da
- ho-hum
- hiss-s-s-s

You might also include gasps, sighs, and groans.

Observation and Evaluation: Does the child discover ways to make body sounds? Can the child find ways to move to these sounds, as well as those in the extended activity?

Curriculum Connectors: Self-expression is one of the first steps in *social studies* for young children, while the creation and interpretation of sound fall under *music*. "How many" is a quantitative concept (*mathematics*).

Echoing Rhythms

. . . .

Clap out short groupings of beats, one at a time, and have the children repeat them. You can choose any beat groupings you like, but you should start as simply as possible (for example, clapping 1-2 at a slow to moderate tempo), counting aloud as you clap.

Once children are familiar with this activity, introduce the most commonly used meters in music. The first of these is 2/4, meaning there are two quarter notes in each measure, or you count to two before beginning again. A quarter note can be likened to a walking step, in that they take approximately the same amount of time to complete. So you will simply count 1-2, 1-2, and so on, at a moderate tempo.

Next is 3/4, or three quarter notes to the measure (clap and count **1**-2-3, **1**-2-3, with the accent on the first beat). The 4/4 meter indicates there are four quarter notes to the measure (clap and count 1-2-3-4). Finally, there is 6/8, indicating six eighth notes to the measure (more like a running step), so you will clap **1**-2-3-4-5-6 at a brisker pace, again with the accent on the first beat.

Extending the Activity: A more challenging method is to clap without counting. When the children are ready, you can invite them to initiate the process. Also, you can try combinations of beat groupings; for example, 1-2, 1-2-3.

Observation and Evaluation: Is the child able to echo the beat groupings? If not, is it due to a problem with hearing, remembering the sequence, or responding in rhythm?

Adding Equipment: Students can respond with rhythm sticks, tambourines, maracas, or hand drums instead of clapping.

Curriculum Connectors: Rhythm, beat groupings, and meter all fall under the heading of *music*; however, rhythm is also essential to the *language arts*. Counting and one-to-one correspondence are components of *mathematics*.

Clapping Names

This is a wonderful activity involving the rhythm of words—more specifically, the children's names.

Beginning with your own name, clap out its rhythm while saying it aloud. For example, my name—Rae Pica (pronounced ray PEE-ka)—would involve three claps, with a pause between the first and the second. The children then echo your name and its rhythm.

Repeat this with all of the children's first names, making sure not to leave anyone out!

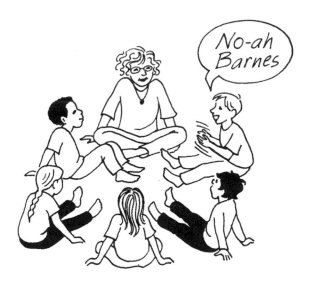

Extending the Activity: When the children are ready, repeat the activity using both first and last names. For a real challenge, include middle names too!

Observation and Evaluation: Is the child able to echo each name? If not, is it due to a problem with hearing, or does the child not understand the concept of one clap per syllable?

Curriculum Connectors: Rhythm is a component of *music* and *language arts*, under which the concept of syllables also falls. One-to-one correspondence (that is, one clap per syllable) brings in *mathematics*.

Pass the Beat

Sit with the children in a circle and clap out a rhythm (for example, 1-2-3-4 at a moderate tempo, or quick-quick-slow-slow). Each child then repeats the rhythm, taking turns around the circle, until the beat is returned to you. The object is to repeat the rhythm *exactly*, keeping an even tempo all the way around the circle.

Extending the Activity: More challenging is to maintain even the interval between each child at a steady rhythm. When the children are ready, they can be invited to lead off with a rhythm of their own.

Observation and Evaluation: Is the child able to repeat the pattern passed with the appropriate rhythm? Can the child initiate a pattern?

Adding Equipment: As with other rhythm activities, these can be performed using rhythm instruments in place of hands.

Curriculum Connectors: Rhythm is a component of both *music* and *language arts*, while counting is part of *mathematics*.

Rain Dance

 "Rain Dance" (Length 2:49)—CD Track 17

This song is in a very definite 4/4 meter, which makes it easy to count, clap, and step to. Experiment with it, asking the children to step forward or to perform a gesture on every one count. Or have them walk four beats and rest four beats, alternately. Even more challenging is to ask them to begin walking in time with the music, changing direction on every one count.

Extending the Activity: This is an excellent activity for enhancing listening skills and provides yet another use for this song.

Begin by sitting and listening to the song, pointing out the flute-like sound made by an instrument called a recorder. This sound is playing more often than not and should be an easy sound for the children to recognize. Then rewind the song and ask the children to move only while the recorder is playing and to freeze when it is not.

Observation and Evaluation: Can the child hear the four beats to the measure? Does the child respond to the one-count? Does the child hear and respond to the recorder?

Adding Equipment: Playing rhythm instruments, such as bells, maracas, drums, or rhythm sticks, can enhance the students' awareness of the 4/4 meter. Be aware that some children are not yet developmentally ready to move and play an instrument simultaneously and will have to do either one or the other.

Curriculum Connectors: Rhythm is a major component of both *music* and *language arts*, as are listening skills. Counting and one-to-one correspondence fall under the content area of *mathematics*.

Common Meters

 "Common Meters" (Length 3:59)—CD Track 18

This song is in four sections, in the four common meters of 2/4, 3/4, 4/4, and 6/8. You and the children should count aloud and clap along with the beat in each section. For example:

- 2/4: Count and clap 1-2, 1-2, and so on.
- 3/4: Count and clap **1**-2-3, **1**-2-3, and so on.
- 4/4: Count and clap 1-2-3-4.
- 6/8: More quickly, count **1**-2-3-4-5-6. Clap along if possible. Otherwise, you can simply raise an arm on every one-count.

Extending the Activity: Can the children step in place on each count? In what other ways can they find to move to each of these sections?

Observation and Evaluation: Can the child differentiate among the meters? Is the child able to count and clap appropriately to each section? Can the child find other ways to respond to the music?

Curriculum Connectors: Rhythm is a component of *music*, while counting and one-to-one correspondence are part of *mathematics*. Active listening is central to *language arts*.

A Not-So-Common Meter

♪ **"A Not-So-Common Meter" (Length 2:00)—CD Track 19**

This song is in a 7/8 meter and has a distinctly different feel. Invite the children to sit and "wiggle" along with it, and/or to show you how the music makes their hands and arms want to move.

Extending the Activity: Once the children are familiar with this less common meter, invite them to stand and to move along with it in any way they wish. Or, if that is too intimidating for some, use it to play a game of Statues, where they move as long as the music is playing and freeze into a statue when you pause it.

Observation and Evaluation: Does the child hear the seven beats? Is the child able to count and clap along with them? Can the child find appropriate ways to move to the song?

Adding Equipment: An alternative is to invite the children to discover how the music makes a prop feel like moving. Possible props include streamers, ribbon sticks, scarves, or hoops.

Curriculum Connectors: Rhythm is central to both *music* and *language arts*, while counting is a component of *mathematics*.

Four Beats to the Measure

 "1-2-3-4" (Length 2:57)—CD Track 20

Here the children are going to discover the variety of ways it is possible to experience four beats to the measure (a 4/4 meter). With you clapping or beating a drum, repeatedly count out four beats (accenting the first count), to which you will ask the children to perform the following:

4 steps	2 steps and 2 claps
3 steps and a clap	1 step and 3 claps

Try this several times. If the children have no problem with it, you can reverse the previous order and pick up the tempo a bit.

Extending the Activity: Although similar to the above, "1-2-3-4" is much more challenging because response time is determined by the rhythm and tempo of the song. The lyrics ask the children to perform the following, and each pattern is repeated before moving on to the next:

- count for 4 beats; repeat
- clap for 4 beats; repeat
- step for 4 beats; repeat
- rest for 4 beats; repeat
- count 2; clap 2; repeat
- clap 2; step 2; repeat
- step 2; rest 2; repeat
- count 1; clap 3; repeat
- clap 1; step 3; repeat
- step 1; rest 3; repeat
- count 3; clap 1; repeat
- clap 3; step 1; repeat
- step 3; rest 1; repeat

Observation and Evaluation: Is the child able to respond appropriately both without and with music? If not, does the problem lie with listening skills or with keeping time?

Curriculum Connectors: Rhythm and meters fall under the heading of *music*, with the counting and patterning components of *mathematics*. Listening skills, required of the extended activity, fall under both music and *language arts*.

Ten Seconds

In this activity the children are going to be limited by the length of time they have to perform a movement or movements.

Explain that you are going to count out ten seconds in your head (so your counting does not influence their movement), telling them when to begin and end moving. During that ten seconds, you want them to show you how many *different* movements it's possible to perform.

Extending the Activity: Next, ask the students to prolong a *single* movement, like raising or lowering an arm, or making a single turn, for ten seconds, this time while you count aloud.

Observation and Evaluation: Does the child demonstrate at least three different movements during the initial activity? Can the child sustain a single movement for ten seconds?

Curriculum Connectors: The concept of time and counting both fall under the heading of *mathematics*.

Let's Swing

 "Swing and Sustain" (Length 1:53)—CD Track 21

Swinging is one of the six qualities of movement, and it takes the form of an arc or a circle around a stationary base. A swing generally requires impulse and momentum, except perhaps when the swinging part is merely released to the force of gravity. Swinging movement can be executed by the body as a whole, by the upper or lower torso alone, and by the head, arms, or legs.

Introduce the children to swinging motion by presenting the following challenges:

- Swing your arms back and forth.
- Show me you can you swing your arms more slowly. More quickly.
- Swing your arms from side to side.
- Swing your head from side to side, as though it were a windshield wiper.
- Swing your arms like an elephant's trunk.
- Show me you can you swing your body as though on a flying trapeze.

Extending the Activity: Use the song to review the quality of swinging movement and introduce the quality of sustained movement. During the "swinging" parts of the music, the children should perform any swinging movements they choose, with all or parts of their bodies. The sustained movement may be more difficult to master, but you can liken it to slow-motion moving, like being in a film played in slow motion. You and the children will easily be able to distinguish one part of the music from the other.

Observation and Evaluation: Is the child able to isolate and swing various parts of the body freely? Does the child differentiate between the swinging and sustained parts of the music? Is the child able to respond appropriately to each?

Adding Equipment: Moving a large chiffon scarf, a streamer, or ribbon stick to the accompaniment of the song can help make the concepts of swinging and sustained movement more visible—and thus more concrete—to the students.

Curriculum Connectors: In addition to the experience with *music*, these activities provide experience with both *science* (the concept of swinging) and *mathematics* (sustained movement is related to the concept of time).

Vibration

 "Vibration" (Length 1:27)—CD Track 22

Use this song to introduce the children to the quality of vibratory movement. You can use the nonvibratory sections, which alternate with vibratory sound, to instruct the children to vibrate in the following ways:

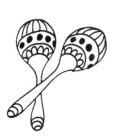

- like a battery-powered toothbrush
- like a leaf shaking in the wind
- like a baby's rattle or a maraca
- as though shivering in the cold

Extending the Activity: Challenge the children to try vibrating individual body parts, such as the head, arms, hands, upper torso, legs, or feet.

Observation and Evaluation: Does the child understand the concept of vibration? Does the child relate to the imagery used? Can the child isolate and vibrate individual body parts?

Adding Equipment: Holding a maraca or another shaking instrument may help demonstrate the concept of vibration.

Curriculum Connectors: Vibration, particularly because it requires a change in muscle tension, falls under the heading of *science*. Using the song adds the element of *music*. The self-expression involved constitutes *social studies*.

Percussion

 "Percussion" (Length 2:06)—CD Track 23

This song introduces the children to the quality of percussive movement. Play the song and ask the children to show you how it makes them feel like moving. If they have trouble with it, you might offer word clues like *jerky*, *jumpy*, or *explosive*.

Extending the Activity: Once they have experimented with moving percussively, using the body as a whole, ask them to try it with different body parts. These can include arms, hands, head, feet, and legs. More challenging would be hips and shoulders.

Observation and Evaluation: Does the child understand the concept of percussive movement? Is the child able to move both the whole body and individual body parts percussively?

Adding Equipment: Playing a hand drum or tambourine while moving to the song may help get the concept of percussion across.

Curriculum Connectors: In addition to the experience with *music*, *science* is also explored here, as percussive movement requires a change in muscle tension.

Suspend and Collapse

. . . .

♪ **"Suspend and Collapse" (Length 1:34)—CD Track 24**

In suspended movement, the body often acts as a base of support, above which one or more parts are temporarily interrupted in their flow of movement. In this case, the movement begins with an impulse, reaches its peak elevation, holds momentarily, and then continues once again. An example would be a swinging arm that stops momentarily overhead before swinging once again. Suspended movement involving the whole body requires control and balance.

Collapsing can be likened to movement that occurs when a puppet is released from its strings or when a building is demolished. A collapse of the human body, however, must always be executed with the necessary control to avoid injury. In addition to the body as a whole, other body parts can collapse, including the head (collapsing to chest, back, shoulder), an arm that has been suspended and then collapses through space, or the upper torso collapsing toward the lower torso.

Invite children to experiment with both qualities of movement. How many ways can they find to suspend and collapse the whole body? How many body parts can they find that can suspend and collapse?

Extending the Activity: This song will provide additional, audible experience with the qualities of suspended and collapsing movement. It is in four parts. During the first part, the children should move or walk in any way they like. The music then suspends, and the children should suspend (halt) their movement also, remembering that suspended movement is different from sustained movement, which keeps on going. A collapsing sound follows, and that is the children's clue to collapse (drop to the floor—safely!). Finally, the music rises, allowing the children time to rise and begin again.

Observation and Evaluation: Does the child understand the concepts of suspended and collapsing movement? Does the child differentiate between suspended and sustained movement? Does the child collapse safely?

Curriculum Connectors: The concepts of suspension and collapse are relative to *science*. Using the song brings in *music*. The word comprehension involved brings in *language arts*.

More Movement Words

As with the Movement Words activities under Educational Gymnastics (page 149), these activities not only provide a review of various movement skills, but they also allow the children to interpret the words in their own ways. For this unit, the words tend to have a greater "emotional" content than those found in Educational Gymnastics.

Begin simply with the words skipping and swinging, telling students what the words are and establishing a signal that indicates it is time to change from one to the other. At the sight, or sound, of the signal, the students perform the specified action in any manner they choose. Repeat this several times, but not so many that the children become bored.

Extending the Activity: Other possible combinations include the following:

- floating and exploding
- scampering and wiggling
- leaping, turning, and dancing
- spinning, flopping, and leaning
- soaring, stamping, and strolling
- tramping, squirming, and swooping

Observation and Evaluation: Does the child interpret the words in an individual way? Is the child able to easily transition from one movement to the next? Does the child respond immediately to the signal?

Curriculum Connectors: These activities involve self-expression, which is part of the first level of *social studies* for young children, and word comprehension and phrases, which is part of *language arts*.

Let's Step-Hop

♪ "Step-Hop" (Length 2:14)—CD Track 25

Like the skip, the step-hop is a combination of a step and a hop. However, with the latter, the step and the hop have the same time value, and the accent is on the step (the hop is accented in the skip). Use a process of guided discovery (convergent problem solving) to help children learn the step-hop. You might issue the following challenges:

- Practice walking forward and in place with short springy steps.
- Hop in place and forward, first on one foot and then the other. Change feet often.
- Make up your own combination of walks and hops, using any number of each. Try it first in place and then moving forward.
- Make up a combination of walks and hops that fits into two counts, slightly accenting the first count.

Validate all responses you see, but the only "correct" response to the final challenge is the step-hop (one step and one hop to a count of 1-2). Once children have it, provide an even 1-2 beat with your hands or a drum and invite the children to practice their newly discovered skill.

Extending the Activity: Challenge children to practice the step-hop to the accompaniment of "Step-Hop." You can use resting spots in the song to challenge them to try the step-hop in the following ways:

- backward
- sideways
- turning
- with arms extended to sides
- with arms folded across chest
- with hands clasped behind the back
- with knee bent and lifted to the front of the hop

The next challenge is to invite children who have mastered the step-hop to pair off, trying it with the following connections:

- inside hands joined
- inside arms linked
- right and left hands joined, with arms crossed
- arms around each other's waists
- inside hands on each other's shoulders
- right hands joined with one partner's arm across the other partner's shoulders and left hands joined in front

Observation and Evaluation: Does the child discover the step-hop through the convergent problem-solving process? If not, is the child able to imitate others who are executing the step? Can the child perform it in a variety of directions and body positions? With a partner?

Curriculum Connectors: Using the song brings in *music*. Also, the step-hop is commonly used in a lot of folk dances; discussion of some of these dances—and their origins—could incorporate *social studies* into the experience. The cooperative aspect of the extension activity is also social studies. Counting and one-to-one correspondence are part of *mathematics*.

A Square Path

. . . .

♪ **"1-2-3-Turn" (Length 1:34)—CD Track 26**

In this activity, the children will move in straight lines but in the shape of squares.

Begin by simply challenging them to make square patterns on the floor with their steps. Then ask them to try turning on every fourth step, to a count of 1-2-3-4.

Extending the Activity: Once the children have practiced this a while, play "1-2-3-Turn," and ask them to try it to the musical accompaniment, always starting on the right foot for count 1. The even 4/4 beat and the recurring sound on count 4 should help. The end result should be that the children walk forward four counts (right-left-right-left), making a quarter turn to the right on count 4.

Observation and Evaluation: Does the child understand the concept of making a square path on the floor? Is the child able to make a square path in sixteen counts, always turning on count 4? Can the child make the square path to the accompaniment of the music?

Adding Equipment: Although involving a more direct approach, you might choose to make the activity easier by placing cutout feet on the floor (four per side) in the shape of a square.

Curriculum Connectors: In addition to the experience with *music*, this activity focuses on squares, a geometrical shape, placing it also under the heading of *mathematics*. Math is also incorporated through the counting and one-to-one correspondence.

Exploring 3/4 Time

♪ **"The 3/4 Song" (Length 1:53)—CD Track 27**

Although the children have experienced a variety of meters at this point—3/4 included—they have focused more often on the even-numbered meters, such as 2/4 and 4/4. In this exercise, the children will focus exclusively on the 3/4 meter in preparation for performing the 3/4-run in later lessons.

"The 3/4 Song" is in two different tempos, first slow and then a bit quicker. Begin by asking the children to sit and clap and count **1-2-3** (with the accent on the 1) along with the song. Other challenges can include stamping the feet **1-2-3** while still sitting (the first count will alternate from right to left foot) and swaying from side to side (the first count will alternate sides).

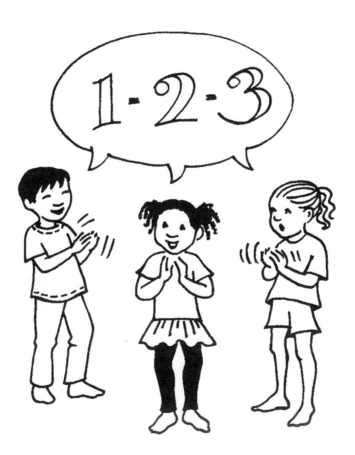

Extending the Activity: The next challenge is to perform a down-up-up motion, while remaining in place, to the 1-2-3. This involves bending the knee on one leg, following by two alternating tiptoes (bend right, tiptoe left, tiptoe right; bend left, and so on).

Observation and Evaluation: Is the child able to count and clap 1-2-3? Can the child stamp 1-2-3 with the feet? Sway 1-2-3? Can the child perform the down-up-up motion in place?

Curriculum Connectors: This activity involves some simple counting and one-to-one correspondence (*mathematics*) and the spatial concepts of up and down (*art*), but it is mostly about moving to a 3/4 meter in *music*.

Zigzagging Pathways

This activity is similar to A Square Path, explored earlier (page 171). This time, however, the children are going to move in zigzags.

Beat out a 3/4 meter at a moderate tempo (**1**-2-3, **1**-2-3). Challenge children to make zigzagging pathways to the accompaniment of your beats. Can they make each line of their zigzags in just three counts?

Extending the Activity: Challenge the children to start their zigzags on the right foot, walking forward on a right diagonal. On count 3, they pivot on the right foot and face diagonally left, beginning on the left foot for the next series of beats. They continue with this zigzag pattern to the right and left, facing a new direction with every first count.

Observation and Evaluation: Does the child understand the concept of zigzagging pathways? Is the child able to create them to the accompaniment of a 3-count?

Curriculum Connectors: The concept of line (zigzagging included) is basic geometry, which falls under the heading of *mathematics* (as does counting). This exercise is also an exploration of the 3/4 meter in *music*.

The 3/4 Run

♪ **"The 3/4 Run" (Length 1:52)—CD Track 28**

Begin by reviewing the down-up-up movement introduced in Exploring 3/4 Time (page 172). Then challenge the children to try the steps while moving forward (that is, they will step right with a bent knee, then rise onto tiptoe for the next two steps on the left and right feet). Having the children say, "Down-up-up," either out loud or to themselves may help them to perform this more successfully.

This activity is conducted without musical accompaniment so each child can attempt to master the steps at whatever tempo is most appropriate. However, when a child has successfully executed the steps, she or he should be challenged to try it at faster tempos until a 3/4 run is being performed. (*Note:* The faster the tempo, the less exaggerated the down-up-up motion will have to be. This is known as a *triplet* in dance terms.)

Extending the Activity: When the children are ready, ask them to perform this movement to the accompaniment of "The 3/4 Run." Once children have mastered this step, challenge them to include their arms. The arms and legs move in opposition: The left arm should swing forward as the right leg steps forward with a bent knee, remaining there through the next two steps on tiptoe; the right arm then swings forward as the left leg bends, and so forth. The accent with the bent knee and arm swing is on the first count.

Observation and Evaluation: Is the child able to execute the down-up-up pattern while moving across the floor? Can the child perform it to the accompaniment of the song, thereby executing a 3/4 run? Is the child able to use the arms in opposition?

Adding Equipment: Once children are executing the 3/4 run with arms in opposition, holding a brightly colored scarf in each hand makes the movement quite visually appealing.

Curriculum Connectors: Down and up are spatial concepts and therefore related to *art* and *mathematics*. Also, while there is some simple counting involved (math), this activity is primarily concerned with moving to a 3/4 meter in *music*.

Making Dances

As a culminating experience for the unit, and possibly the program, challenge students to work with a partner to create their own movement sequences.

Partners should choose one of the three-word sets of More Movement Words (page 168) explored earlier in the unit and perform them in such a way that they create a smooth sequence. They can perform the movements in any order they choose, executing as many repetitions of each as they want, but should not include any extraneous movement in between. They should perform the series they create at least twice through and should include opening and closing poses. Partners can choose to perform in unison or in alternation.

Extending the Activity: More difficult is to play various pieces of music, in different meters, challenging students to match their sequences to the music's rhythm.

Observation and Evaluation: Do the partners link the movements smoothly, as is required by a sequence? Are opening and closing poses included? Do they perform the sequence at least twice through? Can they match their movements to the accompaniment of the chosen music?

Curriculum Connectors: The cooperative nature of the activities falls under the heading of *social studies*. The extended activity incorporates *music*. Also, because the children are now creating movement "sentences," as opposed to phrases, these activities can be linked to *language arts*.

References

AAHPERD (American Alliance for Health, Physical Education, Recreation and Dance). 2004. *Physical Activity for Children: A Statement of Guidelines for Children Ages 5–12*. 2nd ed. Reston, VA: AAHPERD.

Amabile, Teresa M. 1992. *Growing Up Creative: Nurturing a Lifetime of Creativity*. 2nd ed. Buffalo, NY: The Creative Education Foundation Press.

Bar-Or, Oded, John Foreyt, Claude Bouchard, Kelly D. Brownell, William H. Dietz, Eric Ravussin, Arline D. Salbe, Sandy Schwenger, Sachico St. Jeor, and Benjamin Torun. 1998. "Physical Activity, Genetic, and Nutritional Considerations in Childhood Weight Management." *Medicine and Science in Sports and Exercise* 30 (1): 2–10.

Carson, Linda M. 2001. "The 'I Am Learning' Curriculum: Developing a Movement Awareness in Young Children." *Teaching Elementary Physical Education* 12 (5): 9–13. Choosykids.com/CK2resources/eventhost/Day%202 /Body%20Language/The%201%20am%20Moving%20 Curriculum.pdf.

CDC (Centers for Disease Control and Prevention). 2008. "Preventing Diabetes and Its Complications." http://www.cdc.gov/nccdphp/publications/fact sheets/prevention/pdf/diabetes.pdf.

Frostig, Marianne. 1970. *Movement Education: Theory and Practice*. Chicago: Follett Education Corporation.

Gallahue, David L., and Frances Cleland Donnelly. 2003. *Developmental Physical Education for All Children*. 4th ed. Champaign, IL: Human Kinetics.

Garnet, Eva Desca. 1982. *Movement Is Life: A Holistic Approach to Exercise for Older Adults*. Princeton, NJ: Princeton Book Company.

Graham, George. 2008. *Teaching Children Physical Education: Becoming a Master Teacher*. 3rd ed. Champaign, IL: Human Kinetics.

Halsey, Elizabeth, and Lorena Porter. 1970. "Movement Exploration." In *Selected Readings in Movement Education*, edited by Robert T. Sweeney, 71–77. Reading, MA: Addison-Wesley Publishing Company.

Hannaford, Carla. 2005. *Smart Moves: Why Learning Is Not All in Your Head.* 2nd ed. Salt Lake City, UT: Great River Books.

H'Doubler, Margaret Newell. 1925. *The Dance and Its Place in Education.* New York: Harcourt, Brace, and Company.

Kaur, Harsohena, Won S. Choi, Matthew S. Mayo, and Kari Jo Harris. 2003. "Duration of Television Watching Is Associated with Body Mass Index." *Journal of Pediatrics* 143 (4): 506–11. doi: 10.1067/S0022-3476(03)00418-9.

Lewin, Tamar. 2010. "If Your Kids Are Awake, They're Probably Online." *New York Times,* January 20. http://www.nytimes.com/2010/01/20/education /20wired.html.

Mayesky, Mary. 2009. *Creative Activities for Young Children.* 9th ed. Clifton Park, NY: Delmar.

McClenaghan, Bruce A., and David L. Gallahue. 1978. *Fundamental Movement: A Developmental and Remedial Approach.* Philadelphia, PA: W. B. Saunders Company.

McDonough, Patricia. 2009. "Television and Beyond a Kid's Eye View." http:// www.nielsen.com/us/en/newswire/2009/television-and-beyond-a-kids-eye-view.html.

Mosston, Muska, and Sara Ashworth. 1990. *The Spectrum of Teaching Styles: From Command to Discovery.* New York: Longman.

NAEYC (National Association for the Education of Young Children). 2009a. *Developmentally Appropriate Practice in Early Childhood Programs Serving Children from Birth through Age 8.* Position statement. Washington, DC: NAEYC. www.naeyc.org/files/naeyc/file/positions/PSDAP.pdf.

———. 2009b. *NAEYC Standards for Early Childhood Professional Preparation Programs.* Position statement. Washington, DC: NAEYC. http://www.naeyc .org/files/naeyc/file/positions/ProfPrepStandards09.pdf.

Samuelson, Emily. 1981. "Group Development and Socialization through Movement." In *Readings: Developing Arts Programs for Handicapped Students,* edited by Lola H. Kearns, Mary Taylor Ditson, and Bernice Gottschalk Roehner, 53–54. Harrisburg, PA: Arts in Special Education Project of Pennsylvania.

Science Daily. 2010. "Obese Children Show Signs of Heart Disease Typically Seen in Middle-Aged Adults, Researcher Says." http://www.sciencedaily .com/releases/2010/10/101025005835.htm.

Additional Resources

Sources for Ordering Musical Instruments

Childcraft
www.childcrafteducation.com
888-388-3224

Constructive Playthings
www.constructiveplaythings.com
800-448-1412

Lakeshore
www.lakeshorelearning.com
800-428-4414

MMB Music, Inc.
www.mmbmusic.com
314-531-9635

Music in Motion
www.musicmotion.com
800-807-3520

Rhythm Band Instruments
www.rhythmband.com
800-424-4724

Sources for Ordering Equipment and Props

FlagHouse

www.flaghouse.com

800-793-7900

Kaplan Early Learning Company

www.kaplanco.com

800-334-2014

Lakeshore Learning

www.lakeshorelearning.com

800-428-4414

Play with a Purpose

www.pwaponline.com

888-330-1826

US Games

www.usgames.com

800-327-0484

About the Author

Rae Pica is an internationally recognized education consultant specializing in early childhood physical activity. Known for her lively and informative presentations and keynote speeches, she has also consulted for such groups as the *Sesame Street* Research Department, the Head Start Bureau, the Centers for Disease Control and Prevention, the President's Council on Physical Fitness and Sports, Nickelodeon's *Blue's Clues*, Mattel, and state health departments throughout the country. As founder and director of Moving & Learning (www.movingandlearning.com), Rae has been spreading the "movement message" since 1980.

Rae served on the original task force of the National Association for Sport and Physical Education that created *Active Start: A Statement of Physical Activity Guidelines for Children Birth to Age 5*. She is the author of eighteen books, including the three-book Moving & Learning series; *Physical Education for Young Children: Movement ABCs for the Little Ones*; *A Running Start: How Play, Physical Activity, and Free Time Create a Successful Child*, written for the parents of children ages birth to five; and the award-winning *Great Games for Young Children: Over 100 Games to Develop Self-Confidence, Problem-Solving Skills, and Cooperation* and *Jump into Literacy: Active Learning for Preschool Children*.

Additionally, Rae is cofounder of BAM! Radio Network (www.bamradionetwork.com), where she hosts the Internet radio programs *Teacher's Aid* and *Body, Mind, and Child*, and cohosts *NAEYC Radio*, interviewing experts in the fields of education, child development, play research, the neurosciences, and more.